# Educating Children with
# Velo-Cardio-Facial Syndrome

# Genetic Syndromes and Communication Disorders Series

Robert J. Shprintzen, PhD
*Series Editor*

**Waardenburg Syndrome** by Alice Kahn, PhD
**Educating Children with Velo-Cardio-Facial Syndrome**
by Donna Cutler-Landsman, MS, Editor

# Educating Children with Velo-Cardio-Facial Syndrome

*A Volume in the*
*Genetics and Communication Disorders Series*

Donna Cutler-Landsman, MS

*Editor*

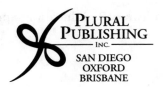

PLURAL
PUBLISHING
INC.
SAN DIEGO
OXFORD
BRISBANE

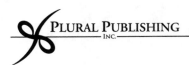

5521 Ruffin Road
San Diego, CA 92123

e-mail: info@pluralpublishing.com
Web site: http://www.pluralpublishing.com

49 Bath Street
Abingdon, Oxfordshire OX14 1EA
United Kingdom

Typeset in 11/13 Garamond by Flanagan's Publishing Services, Inc.
Printed in the United States of America by McNaughton and Gunn

For permission to use material from this text, contact us by
Telephone: (866) 758-7251
Fax: (888) 758-7255
e-mail: permissions@pluralpublishing.com

**Library of Congress Cataloging-in-Publication Data**

Educating children with velo-cardio-facial syndrome / [edited by] Donna
Cutler-Landsman.
     p. ; cm.
 Includes bibliographical references.
 ISBN-13: 978-1-59756-109-9 (soft cover : alk. paper)
 ISBN-10: 1-59756-109-6 (soft cover : alk. paper)
 1.  Genetic disorders in children. 2.  Children with
disabilities–Education. 3.  Face–Abnormalities. 4.  Genetic disorders.
 I. Cutler-Landsman, Donna.
 [DNLM: 1.  DiGeorge Syndrome. 2.  Education, Special–methods.  QS 675
E24 2007]
 RB155.5.E3878 2007
 618.92'0042–dc22
>                                                    2006102379

# Contents

Preface                                                                        vii
  Introduction                                                       viii
  Teacher Awareness Questionnaire                                     ix
Acknowledgments                                                                xiii
Contributors                                                                   xv

**Part I: Scientific Studies and Overview of the Syndrome**                    1

**1**    **Velo-Cardio-Facial Syndrome: Past, Present, and Future**  3
*Robert J. Shprintzen, PhD*

**2**    **Introduction to Education and the Neurocognitive Profile** 15
*Donna Cutler-Landsman, MS, Tony J. Simon, PhD, and
Wendy Kates, PhD*

**3**    **Cognition and the VCFS Brain: The Implications of
Syndrome-Specific Deficits for School Performance**                            39
*Bronwyn Glaser, MA and Stephan Eliez, MD*

**4**    **Psychiatric Disorders and Treatment in
Velo-Cardio-Facial Syndrome**                                                  57
*Doron Gothelf, MD and Merav Burg, MA*

**5**    **Communication in Velo-Cardio-Facial Syndrome**            71
*Karen Golding-Kushner, PhD*

**6**    **Childhood Illness in Velo-Cardio-Facial Syndrome and Its
Impact on School Attendance and Performance**                                  95
*Anne Marie Higgins, RN, FNP, MA*

**Part II: Educational Interventions and Evaluation of
Effective Practices**                                                          113
*Donna Cutler-Landsman, MS*

**7**    **The Early Years: Birth to 3 Programs**                     117

**8**    **Getting Ready for School: Preschool (Ages 3–5)**           119

**9**    **Entering a Formal School Education Program**               135

**10**  **Building the Foundation: Kindergarten through Second Grade (Ages 5–7)**    **143**

**11**  **Gaining Expertise: Upper Elementary Grades Three through Five (Ages 8–11)**    **159**

**12**  **Exploring New Horizons: Middle School (Ages 11–14)**    **179**

**13**  **Choices and Future Goals: High School (Ages 14–18)**    **193**

**14**  **Transition to Adulthood: A Model Program (Ages 18–21)**    **205**

**Conclusion**    **215**

Appendix A: Accommodations    217
Appendix B: Teacher Awareness Questionnaire (Answers)    227
Appendix C: Exercises for Understanding    229

Index    237

# Preface

*I*n 1994, my fourth-grade child was diagnosed with a genetic syndrome called velo-cardio-facial syndrome (also known as VCFS, Shprintzen syndrome, or 22q11 deletion syndrome). After 10 years of speech therapy, occupational services, and various surgeries and interventions, there was finally a name that explained his difficulties. A little blood test called the fluorescence in situ hybridization (FISH) test had just been developed that could positively verify the absence of a piece of DNA on chromosome 22. My husband and I had a genetic explanation and a contact in the United States, Dr. Robert Shprintzen, from New York. No one in Madison, WI, our hometown, knew much at all about the syndrome. In fact, five years earlier a geneticist had looked at our child and his medical history of a heart defect, palate abnormalities, hypotonia, and learning difficulties and screened him for VCFS. He rejected that diagnosis and we spent the next five years searching for answers. Now we had a contact that could help us understand the nature of our child's disability.

Thus began our journey. Eleven years ago, very little was known about the cognitive/learning profile of children with this genetic deletion. No studies were available that focused on how these children learn or what kinds of interventions worked best. What I knew as a parent and teacher of 20 years was that my child was struggling. He learned very differently than others and had trouble remembering directions, understanding math concepts, or telling about what he had read. He was frustrated, I was stressed, and the school was perplexed. What was wrong? Why did techniques typically used for learning disabled students fail with him? Why could he memorize with drill and practice, but have difficulty telling me what he did in school that day? How could he sit through an afternoon of school and fail to learn much of anything?

Since 1994, an enormous amount has been learned about velo-cardio-facial syndrome. Due to the amazing work of the Human Genome Project and scientists at Albert Einstein College of Medicine, the genes that make up the genetic deletion have been identified (Edelmann, Pandela, & Morrow, 1999). Researchers are learning how the genes are expressed and they are beginning to understand why children with the deletion have specific difficulties. Imaging studies from several medical centers such as Upstate Medical University, Stanford University, London, University of California, Irvine, and University of Geneva have uncovered abnormalities in the brains of children and adults with the syndrome. These studies are beginning to explain the reasons for the learning difficulties. Behavior studies have documented particular learning strengths and weaknesses with the VCFS population. Longitudinal studies have highlighted trends that seem to be present and are offering direction for better long-term treatments.

It is estimated that the prevelance of this genetic deletion in the United States and other first world nations is about 1 in 2,000 persons (Robin & Shprintzen, 2005, Shrpintzen, 2005). Yet many children go undiagnosed, schools and teachers remain unaware of the learning profiles of these children, and parents complain that the schools are not preparing their child for any meaningful place in society. A 2005 study conducted by the Stanford University School of Medicine surveyed 53 pediatricians and 69 teachers from northern California as to their knowledge of physical, cognitive, and behavioral features associated with velo-cardio-facial syndrome, fragile X syndrome (X-linked mental retardation), and Down syndrome. The study concluded that the level of awareness of the physical features of VCFS was only 21% among the teachers and that their understanding of the cognitive and behavioral aspects of the syndrome was 8%. Physicians scored only slightly better with only 32% aware of the physical characteristics, 12% knowledgeable of the cognitive profile, and 16% aware of the behavioral issues associated with VCFS (Lee et al., 2005). Clearly, with 92% of teachers surveyed unaware of the learning issues associated with this syndrome, a great deal must be done to educate the general public and medical and learning professionals. It was for this reason that I, along with several other dedicated medical practitioners, decided to write this book. It is our attempt to blend what has been learned in the cognitive science labs with learning theory to give practical advice to all persons who are devoting their time and energy to help a child with VCFS.

The mission of the Velo-Cardio-Facial Educational Foundation, Inc. is to educate the public and professional communities about this syndrome. It is my hope, and the desire of the other contributing authors, that bringing cutting-edge research into the classroom will brighten the lives of the many children with VCFS worldwide who struggle to learn and will serve as a model for educating children with other genetic syndromes. Only with collaboration, experimentation, and reflection will progress occur. We are all continuing to learn.

# INTRODUCTION

This book is divided into two sections. The first deals with the research on VCFS that has been done in several cognitive science labs both in the United States and abroad. Chapters have been contributed by leading VCFS specialists in the areas of speech and language, neurology, psychology, immunology, and cognition. The second section of the text is a practical handbook designed to take the research and apply it to the classroom setting.

While several scientifically controlled studies have been done in neuro-science labs on VCFS and cognition, virtually no research has been done on children with VCFS and teaching interventions. Until recently, very few students were diagnosed with VCFS. There are no specialized schools that group these students together, and those children identified with the syndrome usually do not live in close proximity to each other. Setting up controlled learning environments and testing interventions is a future goal, but it poses many challenges. In the meantime, this book relies on case study data, anecdotal reports from teachers and parents, and educational practice techniques from related studies in special education.

The interventions are grouped according to age level to take into account the unique situations that occur as a child matures. There is, however, a great deal of overlap in appropriate interventions and accommodations. In planning a program for an older child, it will be helpful to read the information for earlier age levels to understand what previous remediation strategies were recommended as well as the section on classroom environment. Many of these early suggestions can also be applied to older students. Also, the back of the book contains appendixes of possible accommodations for specific needs that can be used at any age.

## TEACHER AWARENESS QUESTIONNAIRE

The following questionnaire is a self-test designed to assess your knowledge of the cognitive features associated with Down syndrome, fragile X syndrome, and VCFS. It is adapted from the same questionnaire used by Stanford University School of Medicine to test phenotypic trait awareness of neurogenetic syndromes mentioned earlier (Lee et al., 2005). See how well you do! The answers are in Appendix B.

**Teacher Awareness Questionnaire (Marks of an "X" are correct)**

Please indicate which of the following *cognitive features* are associated with each disorder (*Check all that apply*):

|  | Down syndrome | Fragile X (male) | VCFS |
|---|---|---|---|
| **Arithmetic as a relative weakness, below IQ level** | ☐ | ☐ | ☐ |
| **Relative strength in verbal-based learning** | ☐ | ☐ | ☐ |
| **Ave IQ 70** | ☐ | ☐ | ☐ |
| **Ave IQ 60** | ☐ | ☐ | ☐ |
| **Ave IQ 50** | ☐ | ☐ | ☐ |

| | Down syndrome | Fragile X (male) | VCFS |
|---|---|---|---|
| Deficit in grammar/syntax | ☐ | ☐ | ☐ |
| Short-term memory deficit | ☐ | ☐ | ☐ |
| Perseveration on word, thought, or task | ☐ | ☐ | ☐ |
| Sequencing deficit | ☐ | ☐ | ☐ |
| Expressive language stronger than receptive language (Ability to speak stronger than ability to understand) | ☐ | ☐ | ☐ |

Please indicate which of the following *behavioral features* are associated with each disorder (*Mark with an "X" all that apply*):

| | Down syndrome | Fragile X (male) | VCFS |
|---|---|---|---|
| Attention deficit/hyperactivity | ☐ | ☐ | ☐ |
| Hypernasal speech | ☐ | ☐ | ☐ |
| Gaze avoidance | ☐ | ☐ | ☐ |
| Depression | ☐ | ☐ | ☐ |
| Anxiety | ☐ | ☐ | ☐ |
| Relative preservation of social skills | ☐ | ☐ | ☐ |
| Schizophrenia/bipolar disorder | ☐ | ☐ | ☐ |
| Multiple autistic-like features | ☐ | ☐ | ☐ |
| General happy temperament | ☐ | ☐ | ☐ |
| Tactile defensiveness | ☐ | ☐ | ☐ |

Please indicate which of the following *physical features* are associated with each disorder (*Mark with an "X" all that apply*):

| | Down syndrome | Fragile X (male) | VCFS |
|---|---|---|---|
| Large or prominent ears | ☐ | ☐ | ☐ |
| Vision impairments | ☐ | ☐ | ☐ |
| Cleft palate | ☐ | ☐ | ☐ |
| Delayed motor development | ☐ | ☐ | ☐ |
| Upslanting eyes | ☐ | ☐ | ☐ |
| Hearing problems/deficits | ☐ | ☐ | ☐ |

If you had difficulty with this questionnaire you are not alone. Hopefully, this book will shed some light on how VCFS differs from Down syndrome and fragile X and will offer insight into educational interventions that will make learning more productive for these children.

## REFERENCES

Edelmann, L., Pandela, R. K., & Morrow, B. (1999). Low copy repeats mediate the common 3Mb deletion in velo-cardio-facial syndrome patients on 22q11. *American Journal of Human Genetics, 64*(4),1076–1086.

Lee, T., Blasey, C., Dyer-Friedman, J., Glaser, B., Reiss, A., & Eliez, S. (2005). From research to practice: Pediatrician awareness of phenotypic traits in neurogenetic syndromes. *American Journal on Mental Retardation, 110*(2), 100–106.

Robin N. H., & Shprintzen R. J. (2005) Defining the clinical spectrum of deletion 22q11.2. *Journal of Pediatrics, 147,* 90–96.

Shprintzen R. J. (2005) Velo-cardio-facial syndrome. In S. B. Cassidy & J. Allanson (Eds.), *Management of genetic syndromes* (2nd ed., pp. 615–632). New York: Wiley-Liss.

Shprintzen R. J. (2005) Velo-cardio-facial syndrome. *Progress in Pediatric Cardiology, 20,* 187–193.

# Acknowledgments

*I* would like to express my sincerest gratitude to the contributing authors, professionals and parents of the VCFS Educational Foundation, Inc. and my colleagues at the Middleton Cross Plains Area School District for sharing their support and expertise.

This book is dedicated to my husband, family, and most of all to my son who has taught me patience, understanding, and courage.

# Contributors

**Merav Burg, MA**
The Behavioral Neurogenetics Center
Schneider Children's Medical Center of Israel
Petah Tiqwa, Israel
Psychology Department
Bar Ilan University
Ramat Gan, Israel
*Chapter 4*

**Stephan Eliez, MD**
University of Geneva
Geneva, Switzerland
*Chapter 3*

**Bronwyn Glaser, MA**
Child Psychiatrist and the Middle East Regional Director of the
    Velo-Cardio-Facial Syndrome Educational Foundation, Inc.
Faculty of Medicine
University of Geneva
Geneva, Switzerland
*Chapter 3*

**Doron Gothelf, MD**
Child Psychiatrist and the Middle East Regional Director of the
    Velo-Cardio-Facial Syndrome Educational Foundation, Inc.
The Behavioral Neurogenetics Center
Schneider Children's Medical Center of Israel
Petah Tiqwa, Israel
Sackler Faculty of Medicine
Tel Aviv University
Tel Aviv, Israel
*Chapter 4*

**Anne Marie Higgins, RN, FNP, MA**
Clinical and Research Coordinator
VCFS Center, Upstate Medical University
Syracuse, New York
*Chapter 6*

**Wendy Kates, PhD**
Department of Psychiatry and Program in Neuroscience
State University of New York at Upstate Medical University
Syracuse, New York
*Chapter 2*

**Karen Golding-Kushner, PhD**
Executive Director, VCFS Educational Foundation, Inc.
Private Practice in Speech-Language Pathology
East Brunswick, New Jersey
*Chapter 5*

**Donna Cutler-Landsman, MS**
Middleton-Cross Plains Area School District
Past President of VCFS Educational Foundation, Inc.
Elm Lawn School
Middleton, Wisconsin

**Robert J. Shprintzen, PhD**
Director, Center for the Diagnosis, Treatment, and Study of
   Velo-Cardio-Facial Syndrome
Professor of Otolaryngology
Professor of Pediatrics
Upstate Medical University
Syracuse, New York
*Chapter 1*

**Tony J. Simon PhD**
M.I.N.D. Institute and Department of Psychiatry & Behavioral Sciences
University of California-Davis
Davis, California
*Chapter 2*

# PART I

# Scientific Studies and Overview of the Syndrome

*P*art one of this book is composed of a series of chapters that give an overview of the medical and educational aspects of velo-cardio-facial syndrome. The chapters are written by leading world experts currently involved in scientific research related to the syndrome. The authors have written numerous books and articles on VCFS and have presented their findings at scientific meetings both in the United States and around the world. This section of the book will be particularly helpful to professionals in the fields of speech and language, psychology, education, genetics, and pediatrics, who would like an easy to read summary of the important findings associated with VCFS. It is hoped that this format will allow a treatment plan for children with VCFS that is multi-dimensional and developed with a team philosophy. Only with a deeper understanding of the complexity of the syndrome will better interventions become available. In addition, parents will find this section of the book a helpful guide to better understand and advocate for their child.

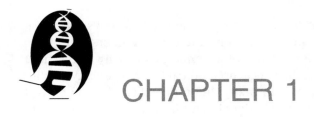

# CHAPTER 1

# Velo-Cardio-Facial Syndrome

## *Past, Present, and Future*

### ROBERT J. SHPRINTZEN, PhD

$M$y first contact with a patient who had the condition I would later call velo-cardio-facial syndrome (VCFS) was in 1974, but it was not until two years later that I would actually start using that name and then another two years later before it was published and made public. Of course, the first patient I saw in 1974 did not strike me as being at all unusual. At the time, I was the director of a large interdisciplinary cleft palate and craniofacial center in New York City and I was seeing hundreds of patients who had hypernasal speech, cleft palate, and other abnormalities of the speech mechanism. Included among those patients were children who had other abnormalities. Some had congenital heart disease, some had cognitive impairments, some had abnormalities of the hands or feet, some had hearing loss, among a large variety of other anomalies. In 1974, these types of associations among anomalies were not well understood, but a new field of study was developing at the time that would change all of that. A group of pioneering clinicians and scientists was studying the relationships between congenital malformations. These pioneers were sometimes referred to as *syndromologists*. Some referred to themselves as *teratologists*, and others called themselves *dysmorphologists*. Although the term dysmorphologist is still used on occasion, today the majority of practitioners who study children with multiple malformations are known as *clinical*

3

*geneticists* or simply *geneticists*. Most clinical geneticists these days are physicians, but in 1974 this was not the case. Among the early pioneers, a number of dental specialists were in the forefront of advances, especially in the field of craniofacial genetics. Because there was no medical board specialty in clinical genetics at that time, people from many different fields of study delved into the process of identifying new disorders in children with multiple anomalies. This early process of syndrome identification was easier at that time because so few syndromes had been identified. In other words, "discovering" previously unknown disorders was much easier when there more disorders that were unknown and when there were so few clinician-scientists taking interest in the field. Today, the field of human genetics is crowded with tens of thousands of specialists who have advanced tests in their diagnostic batteries that were not available (indeed not dreamed of) in those days. As a result, well over 15,000 distinct genetic diseases have been identified, whereas in 1974, the number was a fraction of that.

It is also true that the syndromes that were recognized early on in the study of human genetics were those that had very distinctive characteristics that made them stand out from the general population. Down syndrome, for example, was first identified in the 18th century and described more extensively by John Langdon Haydon Down in the 19th century. VCFS has only recently become recognized. One reason for this delayed recognition is that the large majority of children with VCFS, although characteristic in appearance, are not abnormal in appearance. In other words, children with VCFS resemble each other but do not stick out like a sore thumb (Figure 1–1). Because many of the anomalies are not present at birth (speech, learning, and behavioral disorders), these disorders may not be considered to be congenital anomalies. Another factor is that many children with VCFS have heart malformations that would have been incompatible with survival beyond infancy in the past. Survival following surgical repair of tetralogy of Fallot, interrupted aortic arch, truncus arteriosus, pulmonary atresia, and large ventriculoseptal defects (VSD) is a relatively recent phenomenon and it is likely that many fewer children with VCFS reached adulthood prior to the last three decades.

## VCFS: PAST

The history of the delineation of VCFS as a distinctive syndrome is an interesting study of how advances in medical technology have taken a relatively obscure disorder and made it a focal point of attention by many researchers around the world. As often happens, there is not a single researcher who recognizes the disorder, but there are often many who describe it independently of each other. This is also true for VCFS. Although the name *velo-cardio-facial syndrome* was coined in our 1978 publication (Shprintzen et al., 1978), several other people had already described the syndrome at least in part prior

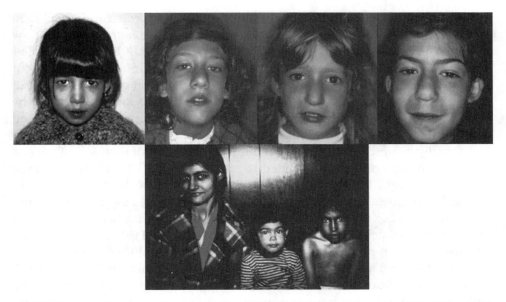

**FIGURE 1–1.** Top row—Four individuals with VCFS. Bottom row—A mother (left) and daughter (right) with VCFS and an uneffective child from the same mother (middle). Courtesy of Dr. Robert Shprintzen.

to that time. The first report that included at least some cases of VCFS was published in a Czechoslovakian medical journal (Sedlaãková, 1955; 1967). Sedlaãková described the association of hypernasal speech with facial hypotonia in a series of cases, and a review of photographs in that article shows that some of the cases clearly had VCFS, although not all did. These articles were descriptions of an interesting phenomenon but were not an attempt to describe a new genetic disorder. Unfortunately, the publication of the article in the Czech language prevented a wider access of the material to the scientific community except in Eastern Europe. In 1968, DiGeorge described congenital absence of the thymus in a series of cases and in that same year, Kretschmer (1968) reported a case he referred to as "DiGeorge's syndrome" that clearly had VCFS. DiGeorge's article was, like that of Sedlaãková, a symptomatic description of a congenital anomaly (thymic aplasia) that has been causally linked to more than one factor, including VCFS, Down syndrome, fetal alcohol effects, and several other chromosome rearrangements. Also in 1968, an article was published that truly delineated the syndrome in significant detail in a large family with multiple affected members. Strong (1968), a pediatric cardiologist, described a mother and three children (plus three other children who did not survive infancy) who clearly had VCFS. The photographs and documentation of the cases were excellent and demonstrated that this was a family with multiple affected individuals with VCFS, but Strong has received little acknowledgment or credit for delineating this syndrome. Interestingly, although Strong did describe cognitive impairment in his report, he did not mention speech disorders. In 1981, I was preparing a paper on VCFS for publication in the journal *Pediatrics* and I gave a draft to one of my residents, Robert W. Marion, M.D., who is now Professor of Pediatrics, Professor of Obstetrics and Gynecology, and Section Chief of Genetics, Department of Pediatrics at the Albert Einstein College of Medicine in New York, to read. He came back to me a few days later and told me that he found the article by Strong and he was convinced that he described the same syndrome. I agreed after reading the article, and I must admit that I was disappointed that Strong had actually beaten me to the punch. I noticed the lack of mention of speech disorders in the article, so I decided to call Dr. Strong. He had moved since the publication of his article and in 1981 he was at the Medical College of Georgia in Augusta. I was able to track him down (not easy in pre-Internet days) and he was very gracious in discussing his work. I asked him if any of the cases he had described had cleft palate. He said (and this is a direct quote because I wrote it down at the time), "Funny you should mention that. None of them had cleft palate, but they all sounded like they had cleft palate." Strong's report clearly delineated the syndrome in a single kindred and essentially established the mode of inheritance as autosomal dominant, something that was subsequently confirmed by our group in 1985 (Williams et al., 1985). In 1976, the first of a series of papers appeared in the Japanese literature describing the same syndrome, albeit with a different name (Kinouchi et al., 1976). In following years, the Japanese would call the disorder *conotruncal anomalies face syndrome*. Because their work was published in Japanese, the English-speaking world largely ignored their contribution until many years later. However, a review of the Japanese publications clearly demonstrates that they were studying the same condition.

Between 1981 and 1992, our group published approximately 20 papers and a number of chapters that described various clinical features of VCFS, including craniofacial structure, speech and language issues, psychological manifestations, inheritance patterns, and eye findings. Then in 1992, two simultaneous findings caused a significant stir in the research community that led to a burst of study of VCFS. The first finding was the association of VCFS with mental illness. The paper that reported this finding was actually a simple letter to the editor in *The American Journal of Medical Genetics* that I submitted early in 1992 that described a number of cases of VCFS who had developed mental illness, the most common diagnosis being schizophrenia, in their teen years (Shprintzen et al., 1992). This report came about not by any specific diligence on my part, but rather by parents of my patients calling to ask if mental illness was a clinical feature of VCFS. The reason why we did not report this until 1992 is that the majority of patients I had been following until that point were young children or infants at the time of referral. It was not until 1992 that many of them reached late adolescence or adulthood. However, prior to that time I did have two patients, one young (14) and one older (61) who had been diagnosed with schizophrenia. At that time we thought the finding was coincidental. Once I had received a number of calls about the onset of mental illness in teen years, we could not ignore the possibility that mental illness was a component of VCFS, so we started recalling many of our patients who were previously discharged from care and began to find a higher rate of mental problems than we could attribute to chance. Later that year, we first came into contact with Peter Scambler in London who was studying children with "DiGeorge syndrome" (the reason for the quotation marks will be explained shortly). He had found that some of these children had deletions of DNA from chromosome 22. In 1985, our research group had reported that "DiGeorge sequence" was a secondary developmental sequence associated with VCFS. Dr. Scambler was curious to know if the cases he had identified represented individuals with VCFS. In order to understand the reason for the quotation marks around DiGeorge syndrome and DiGeorge sequence above, it will be necessary to explain the difference between a syndrome and a sequence (explained below).

---

### Syndrome or Sequence?

A *syndrome* is defined as multiple anomalies in a single individual with all of those anomalies having a single cause. In the case of VCFS, the cause is a deletion of genetic material from chromosome 22 at the q11.2 band. In other words, every patient who has VCFS has this deletion, and everyone who has this deletion has VCFS. A *sequence* is defined as multiple anomalies in a single individual, but these anomalies can all be related back to one of those anomalies that caused a disruption in the normal developmental process. Sequences are not etiologically specific like syndromes. They may have more than one cause. An article on the Web site of The Velo-Cardio-Facial Syndrome Educational Foundation, Inc. (Shprintzen, 1998) describes a sequence in everyday terms that will be useful to the reader. In the case of VCFS, there are several sequences that occur secondary to the syndrome. Two are common (DiGeorge sequence and Robin sequence), and two other sequences, Potter sequence and holoprosencephaly sequence, occur less frequently. DiGeorge sequence is the symptomatic grouping of hypoparathyroidism, thymic aplasia, and congenital heart disease (Robin & Shprintzen, 2005). DiGeorge sequence is found in association with many syndromes, including Down syndrome, Zellweger syndrome, fetal alcohol syndrome, del(10p) syndrome, del(17p) syndrome, and CHARGE syndrome. Also, it is the minority of people with VCFS who have DiGeorge syndrome. Therefore, not everyone who has DiGeorge sequence has a 22q11 deletion and not everyone with a 22q11 deletion has DiGeorge.

We sent a number of blood samples to Dr. Scambler to test for a 22q11 deletion. All of the cases had the clinical diagnosis of VCFS, but half had congenital heart disease and half did not. None met the criteria for DiGeorge, meaning that they did not have hypoparathyroidism. All of them had the deletion and it was therefore concluded that VCFS was caused by a 22q11 deletion (Scambler et al., 1992; Kelly et al., 1993). Other studies followed that confirmed the same findings (Driscoll et al., 1992).

### The Importance of the 1992 Reports

In 1992, the world of molecular genetics was in high gear. New discoveries were coming at a rapid pace, literally on a daily basis. Spurred on during the beginning years of the Human Genome Project, there was a strong push to find genes responsible for mental illness. The nearly simultaneous discovery of mental illness in VCFS linked to a defined region of the human genome in VCFS excited research projects in a number of institutions in the United States and Europe that were later joined by efforts in Israel and Canada. While prior to 1992 there was almost no psychological or psychiatric research involving VCFS other than our 1985 study (Golding-Kushner et al., 1985), today there are many neuropsychologists and psychiatrists who have become interested in VCFS, performed a large body of research, and published a large number of papers in the scientific literature, some of whom are authors in this volume. The reason for the intensification of interest was the notion that if the deletion of DNA from chromosome 22 consistently results in a pattern of behavioral disorders, then genes in that deleted region must play a role in regulating or determining human behavior and mental status. At the time, VCFS was the first firm link between a known genetic region and mental disorders.

## VCFS: PRESENT

VCFS is now the subject of major research efforts around the world. Major efforts in the United States, Canada, Great Britain, Ireland, France, Sweden, Italy, Israel, Japan, Belgium, and Switzerland have been ongoing for a number of years with smaller efforts in a number of other countries. In short, VCFS has moved from obscurity to one of the most important genetic disorders under study today. The emphasis in research has been largely descriptive of the problems associated with the syndrome and how the molecular genetic contributions of the deletion relate to the clinical findings. Probably the largest number of studies has been in the area of psychiatry and cognitive impairment, although there have also been many studies describing physical anomalies. Unfortunately, there has been very little information published on treatment. There has been a small handful of studies focused on surgical outcomes and even fewer studies reporting the treatment of psychiatric illness. Educational issues have received almost no attention at all. It is likely that the relatively recent delineation of VCFS has continued to focus researchers on understanding the syndrome before developing a core of treatment data.

## The Characteristics of VCFS

The intense study of VCFS has resulted in detailed descriptions of the clinical findings in the syndrome. Anything that can be seen, measured, observed, or assessed in any way in a genetic syndrome is called a *phenotype*. VCFS has over 180 known phenotypes. In addition to a wide range of physical malformations, VCFS also has a large number of behavioral and developmental problems. In fact, there isn't an organ system that is spared in VCFS. Although there are so many possible anomalies in VCFS, this does not mean that an affected individual shows all or even most of these anomalies.

## Variable Expression

Variable expression is a phenomenon that certainly keeps the process of syndromic diagnosis interesting. Individuals who have the same genetic alteration or mutation (the appropriate word for a change in DNA composition) may express that change differently. Although the same genetic mutation typically results in a familiar pattern in people who have it, they are not all exactly the same. Actually, essentially all human diseases are like this. For example, some people who get chickenpox have very mild manifestations of infection with the varicella virus. They may have a few pox and a mildly elevated temperature but little else. Others with the same infection can be covered from head to toe with pox, have a very high fever, get an ear infection, and in very severe cases, pneumonia and encephalitis. Genetic diseases are also variable in terms of the number of problems and the severity of the problems within any single affected individual.

When it is reported that there are 188 anomalies associated with VCFS, this refers to a list of all anomalies that have been observed in clinical experience or reported in the scientific literature. No single patient has this number of anomalies; in fact, I am unaware of a single patient who has a majority of these problems. This is simply a list of possible anomalies and serves as a diagnostic guide for clinicians. Another issue is that many of the anomalies are time specific. In other words, feeding problems is a condition of infancy, not adulthood. Conversely, psychosis is most often seen in adult life and rarely in childhood. Therefore, anomalies come and go in the syndrome.

It is also true that no single anomaly in VCFS occurs in 100% of cases. Even common structural anomalies like congenital heart anomalies occur in approximately 75% of cases and palate abnormalities and hypernasal speech in approximately 75%. It is possible that the most common anomalies in VCFS are the educational and behavioral problems. However, even these are not universal and this author is familiar with a number of individuals with VCFS who have above average intellectual performance and no behavioral abnormalities. It is also likely that there are a substantial number of such individuals who are not known to scientists because they are so normal and therefore they are not included in statistical data concerning VCFS.

## Identification

Today, the majority of diagnoses of VCFS are made by pediatric cardiologists because it is recognized that a high percentage of individuals with those anomalies are comprised of individuals with VCFS. For example, over 50% of people born with interrupted aortic arch, type B have VCFS. The majority of people born with truncus arteriosus have VCFS, and over 15% of people with tetralogy of Fallot have VCFS. However, most children with VCFS do not have tetralogy of Fallot, interrupted aortic arch, and truncus arteriosus. The most common heart anomaly in VCFS is ventriculoseptal defect (VSD) (Shprintzen, 2005). Because VSD is the most common congenital heart anomaly, the proportion of cases of VSD that represent people with VCFS is very low, even though VSD is the most commonly found heart defect in VCFS. In many centers, children with tetralogy of Fallot, interrupted aortic arch, truncus arteriosus, and other major heart malformations are screened with fluorescence in situ hybridization (FISH) for a 22q11.2 deletion, but children with less severe anomalies like VSD, atrial septal defect (ASD), and patent ductus arteriosus (PDA) may not be screened. It is also true that many heart abnormalities may escape detection because they are not clinically significant, such as an isolated right-sided aortic arch or minor aortic valve anomalies. Because the majority of cases of VCFS are now being detected based on their heart disease, and the majority of these cases are more severe anomalies, there is an ascertainment bias away from less obvious cases. Therefore, it is true that many children with VCFS go undetected in infancy and reach school age without being identified. This fact emphasizes the need for educators, speech pathologists, and psychologists to be familiar with VCFS and its frequency among children with learning problems, developmental disorders, behavioral problems, and communicative impairment.

Probably the second largest source of identification of children with VCFS is by speech pathologists who are presented with children with cleft palate, submucous cleft palate, or hypernasal speech. Subsequent referral of these patients to cleft palate teams may bring them into contact with clinical geneticists who understand the association of VCFS with cleft palate and hypernasality. Clinical geneticists also identify many cases in infancy when children are detected with structural anomalies other than heart disease that would prompt referral, such as hernias, abnormal appearing ears, severe hypotonia, small lower jaw, spine anomalies, or kidney abnormalities. Other referral sources, although less common, include endocrinologists, immunologists, developmental pediatricians, otolaryngologists, ophthalmologists, neurologists, and gastroenterologists. Only a few cases have been identified initially by psychiatrists, and these cases have primarily been adults with more severe psychiatric illness.

## When to Be Suspicious

For nonmedical people, the question would be, "What would lead me to suggest a referral to a geneticist for evaluation and FISH testing?" Simple probability statistics might help to answer this question. Children with VCFS have multiple anomalies. What would the probability be of a child who does not have a syndrome having multiple anomalies? Let us look at two common human malformations that are present in a high percentage of VCFS cases: VSD and cleft palate. The population prevalence of VSD is approximately 1:500 people (Samanek et al., 1999). The population prevalence of cleft palate (without cleft lip) is approximately 1:3,225 people (Croen et al., 1998). What would the probability be of a child having a cleft palate associated with a VSD? The probability would be 1:500 × 3,225, or 1:1,612,500. The CDC reported just over 4,000,000 births in the United States in 2004, meaning that we would expect to see no more than 3 children born with the association of cleft palate and VSD in that year. However, in 2004, I saw more children born with that association in just one month in the metropolitan area of Syracuse (population of approximately 736,000 in 2004) with fewer than 15,000 births for the region. Therefore, the frequency of this association is far more than chance would predict; one would expect thousands of births in the United States with this association based on my Syracuse experience . . . not just 3 or 4. The implication is that the association of VSD and cleft palate is not a chance occurrence in almost all cases because both anomalies are caused by the same basic etiology, usually genetic. These probabilities relate to the association of two common structural anomalies, but behavioral anomalies are no different. A subnormal IQ or learning disabilities are regarded as congenital anomalies, and their presence in association with structural malformation only increases the probability that there is a syndromic association. For example, mental retardation occurs in 2 to 3% of the general population. Therefore, the prevalence of a chance association of VSD, cleft palate, and mental retardation would be 1:400 × 3,225 × 50, or 1:64,500,000. If this were the prevalence of these features occurring together by chance, the association would be so rare as to be seen only once every other decade. However, all three of these findings (plus many more) are commonly seen in a number of syndromes, including VCFS, Down syndrome, Kabuki syndrome, fetal alcohol syndrome, and a number of other multiple anomaly disorders. Therefore, if a teacher, speech pathologist, psychologist, or any other professional has contact with a child who has two or more major anomalies, it is legitimate to inquire if the child was seen by a geneticist. If the child has not been evaluated by a geneticist, the suggestion should be made to obtain one. It is not necessary to have a specific suspicion about a particular diagnosis. A child with multiple anomalies warrants a genetic evaluation no matter what the potential diagnosis. Avoiding such a referral not only places the child at risk; it also places the family's reproductive future at risk should the condition be genetic.

## VCFS: THE FUTURE

With the burst of activity associated with VCFS, what are the goals of this research? It may seem unnecessary to say that the goal is improved patient care because this is obviously the reason why scientists study all diseases. Beyond the obvious, the goal would be to avoid symptomatic treatment and develop the ability to avoid the development of problems in the first place. Therefore, researchers are focusing on how the genomic error in VCFS causes the many anomalies seen in the syndrome. Once the basic biology of congenital heart anomalies, palate malformations, immune disorders, learning problems, and mental illness is understood, the goal would be to intercept them, whether that interception is in utero or postnatal. Although we may have difficulty in grasping this concept today, it is clear that the rapid advance of the study of genomic diseases will take us there. All aspects of medicine may be called to the fore to help with this process, including early identification, gene therapy, medicines, and new surgical techniques.

Perhaps the next major advance will be in the realm of diagnosis. Today, whole genome chips are becoming available that will allow the identification of genetic diseases with a small amount of blood that will allow a DNA analysis with a microchip. Today in the year 2006, these chips are very expensive (over $1,000) and are being used almost exclusively for research, including VCFS research at our Center. However, as the technology becomes more commonplace and medical manufacturers develop large-scale production, the price will drop precipitously and cost will not be a factor.

Finally, there is the "I don't believe it" factor. When I first began studying VCFS in the 1970s, if you had told me that we would know of the microdeletion that causes the syndrome, I would have said, "I don't believe it." If in the 1980s you told me we would know of all of the genes that are deleted in VCFS, I would have said the same thing. If in the early 1990s you had told me that we would understand the mechanism of the deletion, my eyes would have opened even wider with the same declaration. Although I don't know what the next "I don't believe it" will be, I am confident that one is coming. Although I have a very good imagination, the science of genomics is so intense with so many excellent minds pursuing it, I am certain that surprises, very pleasant ones, are on the way. Be optimistic.

# REFERENCES

Croen, L. A., Shaw, G. M., Wasserman, C. R., & Tolarova, M. M. (1998). Racial and ethnic variations in the prevalence of orofacial clefts in California, 1983–1992. *American Journal of Medical Genetics, 79,* 42–47.

DiGeorge, A. M. (1968). Congenital absence of the thymus and its immunologic consequences: Concurrence with congenital hypoparathyroidism. *Birth Defects Original Article Series, 4*(1), 116–121.

Driscoll, D. A., Spinner, N. B., Budarf, M. L., McDonald-McGinn, D. M., Zackai, E. H., Goldberg, R. B., et al. (1992). Deletions and microdeletions of 22q11.2 in velo-cardio-facial syndrome. *American Journal of Medical Genetics, 44,* 261–268.

Goldberg, R., Marion, R., Borderon, M., Wiznia, A., & Shprintzen, R. J. (1985). Phenotypic overlap between velo-cardio-facial syndrome and the DiGeorge sequence. *American Journal of Human Genetics, 37,* A54.

Golding-Kushner, K., Weller, G., & Shprintzen, R. J. (1985). Velo-cardio-facial syndrome: Language and psychological profiles. *Journal of Craniofacial Genetics and Developmental Biology, 5,* 259–266.

Kelly, D., Goldberg, R., Wilson, D., Lindsay, E., Carey, A., Goodship, J., et al. (1993). Velo-cardio-facial syndrome associated with haplo-insufficiency of genes at chromosome 22q11. *American Journal of Medical Genetics, 45,* 308–312.

Kinouchi, A., Mori, K., Ando, M., & Takao, A. (1976). Facial appearance of patients with conotruncal anomalies. *Pediatrics Japan 17,* 84–87.

Kretschmer, R., Say, B., Brown, D., & Rosen, F. S. (1968). Congenital aplasia of the thymus gland (DiGeorge's syndrome). *New England Journal of Medicine, 279,* 1295–1301.

Robin, N. H., & Shprintzen, R. J. (2005). Defining the clinical spectrum of deletion 22q11.2. *Journal of Pediatrics, 147,* 90–96.

Samanek, M., & Voriskova, M. ( 1999). Congenital heart disease among 815,569 children born between 1980 and 1990 and their 15 year survival: A prospective Bohemia survival study. *Pediatric Cardiology, 20,* 411–417.

Scambler, P. J., Kelly, D., Lindsay, E., Williamson, R., Goldberg, R., Shprintzen, R. J., et al. (1992). Velo-cardio-facial syndrome associated with chromosome 22 deletions encompassing the DiGeorge locus. *Lancet 339,* 1138–1139.

Sedlaãková, E. (1955). The syndrome of the congenitally shortening of the soft palate. *Cas Lek Ces 94,* 1304–1307.

Sedlaãková, E. (1967). The syndrome of the congenitally shortened velum: The dual innervation of the soft palate. *Folia Phoniatrica 19,* 441–450.

Shprintzen, R. J. (1998). The name game. Newsletter of the *VCFS Educational Foundation,* 1998, Spring.

Shprintzen, R. J., Goldberg, R., Golding-Kushner, K. J., & Marion, R. (1992). Late-onset psychosis in the velo-cardio-facial syndrome. *American Journal of Medical Genetics, 42,* 141–142.

Shprintzen, R. J., Goldberg, R. B., Lewin, M. L., Sidoti, E. J., Berkman, M. D., Argamaso, R. V., et al. (1978). A new syndrome involving cleft palate, cardiac anomalies, typical facies, and learning disabilities: Velo-cardio-facial syndrome. *Cleft Palate Journal, 15,* 56–62.

Shprintzen, R. J., Goldberg, R., Young, D., & Wolford, L. (1981). The velo-cardio-facial syndrome: A clinical and genetic analysis. *Pediatrics, 67,* 167–172.

Strong, W. B. (1968). Familial syndrome of right-sided aortic arch, mental deficiency, and facial dysmorphism. *Journal of Pediatrics, 73,* 882–888.

Williams, M. A., Shprintzen, R. J., & Goldberg, R. B. (1985). Male-to-male transmission of the velo-cardio-facial syndrome: A case report and review of 60 cases. *Journal of Craniofacial Genetics and Developmental Biology, 5,* 175–180.

# CHAPTER 2

# Introduction to Education and the Neurocognitive Profile

DONNA CUTLER-LANDSMAN, MS
TONY J. SIMON, PhD
WENDY KATES, PhD

*V*irtually all children with a neurodevelopmental disability will have challenges learning as quickly or efficiently as a typically developing child. Children with the 22q11.2 deletion often present with significant developmental delays in the speech, cognition, and motor domains. Most children with VCFS will require some type of special education services. Many will need assistance throughout their school years in the areas of academic growth, social relationships, and life skills development. This chapter will explore the research studies that have been completed with children diagnosed with the 22q11 deletion. From these studies, a clearer picture will emerge of a typical profile of strengths and weaknesses in intellectual and achievement domains. These findings will help determine whether a typical child with VCFS has the ability to process information and complete academic tasks. Again, it should be emphasized that there is wide variability within the syndrome, and every child must be carefully screened to create his or her individual profile. Nonetheless, there seem to be some areas of impairment that are found in the majority of children with VCFS assessed.

There have been two main avenues that have been explored to test mental functioning of individuals with VCFS. They are neuropsychological testing and cognitive experimentation studies. This chapter will deal with the neuropsychological testing results and a second chapter will be devoted to brain imaging and cognitive experimentation studies. Neuropsychological testing is the widely accepted approach that schools use to determine if a child is in need of special education services. A battery of standardized tests that focus on the intellectual, academic, and behavior domains is administered. The tests are given by evaluators who are trained to closely follow test protocol and who are skilled in interpreting the results. Standardized test scores are normed in respect to the general population at the same chronological age. From this, standard scores and percentile ranges are generated. Schools use these scores to determine if children are developing at a rate significantly below or above what would be expected for their age and grade level. Test scores can be compared both between individual students and within the child to see if any patterns of strengths or weaknesses occur. Often this battery of tests is administered within a short time period, such as over one to two sessions. This can be advantageous in that a single testing session can generate a great deal of information. The drawback, however, is that the testing session is just a snapshot of how the child performs on a daily basis. With VCFS or other health-impaired children, caution should be taken regarding extended test taking sessions. Since these students tire easily and often have chronic health issues, prolonged testing periods may not be reliable. A more accurate assessment of ability would be gained from testing sessions spread over several days, observations of parents and teachers, and day-to-day performance in the classroom.

While neuropsychological testing can offer assistance with planning an individual education plan, the results are merely descriptive and contribute little in terms of understanding the reasons for the underlying cognitive and neurobiological impairments. The tests can indicate a student has strengths and weaknesses in particular areas, but they really cannot explain the mental processes being used, the brain circuits activated, or the neurotransmitters involved. A small but growing number of cognitive experimentation studies have been done to try to begin to answer these questions. The results of these experiments will be discussed in the next chapter, Cognition and the VCFS Brain.

## GENERAL COGNITIVE ABILITY

The range of neuropsychological impairments seen in VCFS is variable, but numerous studies have identified a pattern of difficulties that seems to be consistent across the VCFS population. On measures of general intelligence or IQ, children with VCFS score lower than would be predicted by their chronological age and lower also than unaffected family members such as parents and siblings. Studies have consistently measured IQ in the low average to borderline range. While normal IQ is considered 100 + 15 standard deviation points, verbal IQ for children with VCFS typically ranges from 75 to 80 and performance (nonverbal IQ) from 70 to 75 (Moss, Batshaw, Solot, Gerdes, McDonald-McGinn, et. al, 1999). A longitudinal study of 103 children from 4 to 16 years in age found the mean total IQ of the group to be 73, with scores ranging from 50 to 109 The study found no difference in IQ in children with the concurrent diagnosis of either a heart defect or ADD. The study did find, however, that children who had a diagnosis of autism as well as VCFS had significantly lower IQ scores. This study also looked at whether there was a difference in IQ levels for children born to parents who did not have the VCFS deletion (de novo) compared to children born to a parent who also had VCFS (familial). In this study 93 children were de novo compared to 10 who were born to an affected parent. The average IQ for the de novo group was 74 compared to 63 for the familial group. While there is likely to be some genetic component to the measured intellectual abilities, it is much harder for children to excel intellectually and academically in a home where at least one parent's intellectual capacities are also impaired.

There is some evidence to suggest a drop in IQ scores from the preschool level of the mid 80s to the mid 70s in elementary school years (Golding-Kushner, Weller, & Shprintzen, 1985; Shprintzen, 2000). The former scores were obtained using the Leiter and Stanford Binet tests and the second set of scores used the Wechsler. Golding-Kushner et al. (1985) suggested that this reduction could be due to the nature of the tests administered rather than a drop in global intelligence. The Wechsler test for older children involves more abstract reasoning and higher order thinking skills, an area of relative weakness for the VCFS population. A 2001 study of 112 VCFS children under the age of 6 used the Wechsler Preschool and Primary Scale of Intelligence (WPPSI-R) and the Bayley Scale to test for IQ (Gerdes, Solot, Wang, McDonald-McGinn, & Zackai, 2001). This study found 34% of the preschool children tested in the average range with IQ scores in the average range (FSIQ > 85), 32% in the mildly delayed range (FSIQ 70–84), and 33% in the significantly delayed range (FSIQ < 70). A longitudinal study out of Stanford found a drop in verbal IQ as children mature with declines in the areas of similarities, vocabulary, and comprehension. This study also marked a decline in expressive language abilities (Gothelf et al., 2005).

Several studies have suggested that VCFS children have more developed verbal than nonverbal abilities. In one study of 33 children with VCFS, Moss and colleagues found that full scale IQ was 71.2 ± 12.8 (mean ± standard deviation), verbal IQ was 77.5 ± 12.8 (mean ± standard deviation) and performance IQ was 69.1 ± 12.0 (Moss et al., 1999). This pattern of performance IQ being significantly higher than verbal IQ, indicative of a nonverbal learning disability, seems to be true for most VCFS children, but not all (Campbell & Swillen, 2005; Moss et al., 1999). Another study of 103 children with VCFS found the average verbal IQ to be 78 compared to a 72 performance IQ. In addition, 3 out of 4 children tested had a verbal IQ higher than their perform- ance IQ and 22% of these children had discrepancies over 15 IQ points (Swillen, 2006).

Consistently, however, neuropsychological or psychometric test results show general intelligence is lower than average with most IQ scores in the 70 to 85 range. Thus, most children with VCFS will have difficulties across both performance and verbal domains in comparison to typically developing peers.

There are also preliminary indications that there may be a difference in cognitive functioning between boys and girls. A study of 90 VCFS children (50 boys and 40 girls) found that boys with VCFS were more cognitively impaired than girls (Antshel, AbdulSabur, Roizen, Fremont, & Kates, 2005). Their aver- age IQ scores on the WISC III were 68.9 ± 12.8 for the boys and 76.3 ± 11.7 for the girls. In addition, this study noted a negative association between age and cognitive functioning with girls and VCFS, in that scores did not keep up with the expected improvement with age, but this was not the case with boys. This study also found that boys with VCFS scored significantly lower than girls with VCFS on measures of communication, daily living skills, and socialization on the Vineland Adaptive Behavior Scale. In addition, boys also scored significantly lower than girls on the Wechsler Individual Achievement Test 2 in the areas of reading, math, written language, and oral language. It should be noted that although girls in this study did better than boys, their scores were still in the low average range and at levels that would necessitate special education intervention. The 2006 study by Swillen found no difference between IQs of males versus females, but another study (Niklasson, Rasmussen, Oskarsdottir, & Gillberg, 2006) of 100 children with VCFS showed girls outscoring boys with average IQ scores of 74 compared to 65 for the boys. Another large study (Kates, 2006) of 160 children aged 9–12 also showed a higher average IQ for girls at 75.95 than for boys at 68.9.

## MATHEMATICS

Academic deficits are very common in VCFS and are most pronounced in math. This can be due to a combination of difficulty with visual spatial tasks, working memory impairments, and weaknesses in problem solving abilities. An early study using the Wide Range Achievement Test (WRAT) demonstrated that math scores among 6–11 year olds with VCFS ranged from 81 to 90 (pop- ulation mean = 100, SD =10) and from 74 to 86 among affected adolescents (Golding-Kushner et al., 1985). Many more recent studies have found results consistent with this initial report. The weaknesses in math seem particularly pronounced in the areas of abstract reasoning, converting language into mathematical expressions, telling time, using money, and problem solving (Kok & Solman, 1995). Another study of 33 individuals with VCFS found lower composite math achievement scores in comparison to scores of reading and spelling (Moss et al., 1999). A recent study looked at 27 children with VCFS aged 6 to 12 and found 19 out of 25 performed at an abnormally low level on at least one of the math variables tested (De Smedt et al., 2006). The children in this study could read numbers accurately and could retrieve number facts, but had difficulty with such things as understanding number magnitude, identifying and ignoring irrelevant information in story problems, and with accuracy on multiplication with more than single-digit numbers. The older students in this study also worked more slowly than age matched controls, which may have educational implications. A more comprehensive discussion on the math deficits associated with VCFS can be found in the next chapter.

## READING

In a study of 50 children with VCFS aged 6–17, reading, decoding, and phonological abilities were found to be stronger than comprehension skills (Woodin et al., 2001). Many children with VCFS reportedly do reasonably well in early elementary school where the emphasis is on learning to read words. By the end of third grade, however, they begin to experience much more difficulty. Accordingly, children with VCFS seem to be more adept at "learning to read" than at "reading to learn." This is thought to be due to the shift from learning skills that are basic and concrete to mastering more abstract, integrated concepts.

## LANGUAGE

Language development can be slow and this may be due to at least two independent causes. One is palate abnormalities and the other is a probable, but as yet unidentified, neural basis. Numerous studies have documented language impairment in VCFS during infancy, preschool, and through to adulthood (Golding-Kushner et al., 1985; Moss et al., 1999; Gerdes et al., 1999; Scherer, D'Antonio, & Kalbfleisch, 1999). Early surgery and speech therapy can address articulation difficulties, but communication deficits can persist indefinitely. Some researchers have found that receptive language usually tends to be more developed than expressive (Moss et al., 1999). There is one study of a group of 27 VCFS children and adolescents, however, which reported the opposite results. Those researchers found stronger expressive than receptive language skills (Glaser et al., 2002). The authors suggest that expressive language may have improved due to speech therapy and/or that as children mature, receptive language abilities require more complex and abstract thinking, an area of weakness for VCFS children. This particular study included several older children and this may indicate a trend for a reversal of language strengths as a child matures. The authors also noted that the children and young adults in this study still performed more poorly on standardized tests of language ability than would have been predicted from their verbal IQ scores. Another large study by Solot et al. also supported the higher expressive than receptive scores for older children (Solot et al., 2001). This study separated 79 VCFS children into two groups, preschool (7–66 months) and school aged (5–16 years). The receptive language scores were higher than expressive for the preschoolers, but the opposite pattern was true for the older children.

Either way, educators should recognize that VCFS children have communication difficulties that severely impact their ability to function in a regular classroom with typically developing peers. In later school years, as expressive language skills improve, teachers may not immediately recognize the need for language intervention. The growth in expressive language abilities may mask the still present receptive language impairments that can be very problematic in discussion/lecture-oriented upper grade courses. Many children with VCFS also continue to have persistent pragmatic language impairments (i.e., language that deals with practical day-to-day communication) that interfere with social interactions as they mature (Glaser et al., 2002). These skills will need additional attention by speech therapists and educators. Specific impairments include difficulty with small talk and with carrying on "to and fro" casual conversations (Vorstman et al., 2006). This researcher also reported that children with VCFS tend to follow their own chain of thought rather than pick up on others' statements as an avenue to explore others' ideas. Many avoid looking at the speaker and may also engage in parallel play rather than become involved with the group (Vorstman, 2006, personal communication). The ability to communicate well enough to convey detailed accounts of events, to request assistance in complicated situations, or to participate in technical conversations may continue into adulthood and has a more profound effect as the child with VCFS reaches adolescence.

Written language skills, including learning grammatical rules and spelling, seem to be relatively strong in comparison to spoken language, but still lag behind same-age peers. Poor fine motor control, however, can make writing laborious and can affect classroom performance.

## MOTOR ABILITIES

Many children with VCFS have hypotonia or low muscle tone. This can impact their ability in both the fine and gross motor domains, especially in tasks that require quick movements or reactions. Many demonstrate difficulty manipulating crayons and pencils, cutting with scissors, or manipulating small items. In a 2005 study by Sobin et al., scores for VCFS children in the areas of motor dexterity (finger tapping), kinesthetic/tactile awareness (imitating hand positions), and graphomotor control (visuomotor precision) from the NEPSY battery were all at least one standard deviation below average (Sobin, et al. 2005). However, it is quite likely that these impairments were not totally the result of motor impairments but may also have been partly due to problems with the mental representation of space and time (known as spatiotemporal representations) that are used to control such movements. This issue is dealt with in more detail in the following chapter. In another study of motor development using the Peabody Development of Motor Skills and the Bruininks-Oseretsky Test of Motor Proficiency, children with VCFS aged 6–12 presented a significant motor delay in both the fine and gross motor domains (Van Aken et al., 2006). The children tested had trouble with skills such as walking on a straight line, hopping on one foot, and placing objects in a box. These motor deficits can impact the ability of these children to perform many tasks in the classroom with speed and accuracy.

## MEMORY

Memory skills can be both a strength and a weakness for VCFS youngsters. Rote verbal memory, or the ability to repeat back a list of items after a delay, was found to be age appropriate in a small study of school-age children (Swillen et al., 1999). In another study (Woodin et al., 2001), 50 children aged 7 to 16 years were tested on their ability to remember lists of unrelated words and of words in specific categories. Even though 62% of the children had IQs in the borderline to moderately deficient range, 72% of the group scored in the low average to very superior range for these memory tasks. Other studies (Wang, Woodin, Kreps-Falk, & Moss, 2000; Bearden et al., 2001) also found a strength in the area of memory for lists or objects.

More complex memory tasks, however, present significant difficulties for VCFS children. Woodin et al. (2001) found that VCFS children demonstrated considerable weakness with delayed recall of story details. Their test subjects scored in the borderline range. These same children also had great difficulty with memory for visual spatial forms. Another study involving a larger sample also showed below average performance for spatial memory tasks (Wang et al., 2000). In addition, Bearden et al. (2001) found that the ability to remember was dependent on the nature of the information to be recalled. The subjects in this study had an easier time remembering the shape of objects than they did the location of dots on a grid. Thus, for example, it might be best to use landmarks and verbal cues for a route rather than to use directional or map-based instructions.

## EXECUTIVE FUNCTION AND WORKING MEMORY

While there have not been a lot of neuropsychological studies in this area, there have been a few researchers that have found significant impairments in this area. Woodin et al. (2001) noted significant impairment in the B subtest of the trail making test on the Wechsler Intelligence Scale for Children (WISC III) when compared to the A subtest. This A subtest requires the child to connect with a pencil a series of locations labeled A, B, C or 1, 2, 3. The B subtest adds complexity to the task by requiring the child to not only connect the locations assigned to the letters in order, but also to alternate between letters and numbers. The letter A connects to 1, B to 2, C to 3, and so on. This additional load on working memory was problematic for the VCFS children tested. Sobin, et al. (2005) also found working memory, or the ability to not only store information but to manipulate it, was an area of specific weakness for VCFS children.

## ATTENTION

Attention is, in fact, a very complex construct and refers to a wide range of cognitive operations involved with the selection of important information from a complex environment, with the inhibition or "ignoring" of less relevant information, and with the apportionment of mental effort for what is often referred to as "cognitive control." Issues relating to the selection of relevant information and its role in tasks like arithmetic are dealt with in the following chapter. The cognitive control aspect is strongly related to the Executive Function and Working Memory section that preceded this one. The task of inhibiting irrelevant information and related aspects of distractibility are ones of great concern for children with VCFS, and this is what is referred to most often when the topic of attention is spoken of. Because of these problems attention deficit disorder is a common diagnosis for VCFS children. More information will be covered regarding this area in the next two chapters. Neuropsychological testing can give some general insight into whether attention issues are affecting performance. Woodin et al. (Woodin et al., 2001) found that the 50 VCFS children tested scored significantly lower on the Freedom from Distractibility index on the WISC III than on the Verbal Comprehension Index on that test. Sobin et al. (2005) also found VCFS children had an area of weakness in Visual Attention).

## COMPREHENSION

As has been discussed elsewhere, children with VCFS have considerable trouble with the task of comprehension. Roughly, this refers to the integration of various pieces of information that have been gathered from listening, reading, or seeing and assembling them into a meaningful structure, such as a set of directions. Children with VCFS can often successfully read a set of instructions with few errors but still be unable to follow any of them at the end of the process. This topic has received little or no scientific investigation until now and it should become a high priority. However, based on what is already known about information processing problems in children with VCFS, one likely source of the problem relates to the issue of attention since a key component of comprehending is being able to pick out the relevant details from a flow of information and determining the critical relationships between them. For example, if one read a story about a person walking down a leafy street on a sunny day and taking the second right turn after the mailbox in order to reach a store and then the reader's task was to explain how to reach the store, one would ignore details of the weather and the leaves but pay attention to the order of the streets and their relation to the mailbox. The storage of information in working memory so that it can be integrated with information that comes much later in the story is important also. Finally, being able to store information in long-term memory is also likely to be an issue because often parents seem to complain that their child can know how to follow instructions one day and no longer remember how to do the same thing a week later.

## BEHAVIORAL AND PSYCHIATRIC ISSUES

Several studies have also identified psychiatric and behavioral phenotypes. VCFS children are highly vulnerable to developing social deficits and psychiatric difficulties that impact learning and functioning. Attention deficit disorder, anxiety, and mood instability are common. Overactivity, impulsivity, shyness, and disinhibition have also been reported in the literature. As a child matures, there tends to be a progression to more emotional problems. Repeated school failures can be extremely damaging to children with this syndrome. Therefore, parents, physicians, and professionals must be proactive to educate the public about this syndrome. Some research identifies over 60% of adults with VCFS diagnosed with some type of psychiatric problem (Papolos et al., 1996). A smaller but still significant number of adults have a more severe mental illness such as rapid cycling bipolar disorder or schizophrenia. The chapter on psychiatric difficulties will go into this area in more detail.

Some children with VCFS display a marked difficulty in the social arena. Some are shy and withdrawn, have difficulty interacting with others, and display limited facial expressions (Gerdes et al., 1999; Niklasson et al., 2002). A 2005 study of 98 children with the 22q11.2 deletion assessed the presence of autistic spectrum disorder as a comorbid condition in this population (Fine et al., 2005). Results of this study found over 20% of the children were exhibiting significant levels of autism spectrum symptoms. A similar result was found in a study out of Syracuse University that found 20% of the VCFS children tested had autism and another 20% showed autisticlike behaviors (Kates, 2006). The label of autism has not typically been associated with a VCFS diagnosis in the literature and this is a controversial area that warrants additional careful study. School personnel, however, are urged to look at the area of social functioning when testing a student with VCFS for special services. Educational methods used for students with autistic spectrum disorders may also be helpful when planning a program for an individual with VCFS.

## LONGITUDINAL STUDIES AND ADULT OUTCOMES

Several longitudinal studies are currently in progress that will provide critical information about the cognitive and psychiatric trajectories of children with VCFS as they move into adulthood. Very few of those studies have reached completion at this time, however. As noted above, for example, one longitudinal study found a drop in verbal IQ as children mature with declines in the areas of similarities, vocabulary, and comprehension (Gothelf et al., 2005). Primarily, however, we must rely on studies that focus on adults only in order to understand the challenges that face adults with VCFS.

Studies on the neuropsychological profiles of adults with VCFS are relatively scarce; however, they do suggest that the cognitive strengths and weaknesses of adults are similar to those of children. In 2002, Henry et al. reported cases of adults with VCFS who had significant impairments in visuoperceptual ability, problem solving, planning, and abstract thinking (Henry, van Amelsvoort, Morris et al., 2002). Similarly, preliminary data from another study (Antshel et al., 2006) suggest that young adults with VCFS continue to exhibit deficits in executive function and memory. Impairments in auditory memory in particular appear to be disproportionate to overall intellectual function in young adults with VCFS (Antshel et al., 2006). Impairments in problem solving and auditory memory may pose specific challenges for adults with VCFS in a work environment.

Moreover, these preliminary data suggest that the adaptive living skills of young adults with VCFS continue to be delayed. Although motor skills, social communication skills, and daily living skills are commensurate with overall intellectual function, it appears that several community living skills are disproportionately impaired in VCFS-affected young adults (Antshel et al., 2006). Studies with young adults suggest that, whereas many VCFS adults in their 20s have developed adaptive skills in the workplace and in the community (around which they can navigate fairly independently), they continue to exhibit significant impairments in the management of both time and money. Therefore, they will continue to require support and intensive training in this domain.

The following vignettes illustrate the variability in functioning that young adults with VCFS display despite comparability in overall intellectual function and psychiatric status.

## Case Study 1

J. is a 25-year-old female with a full scale IQ of 78 (verbal IQ, 76; performance IQ, 84). Her adaptive living skills are commensurate with her IQ, although she acknowledges that she has difficulties in managing money and adapting to some of the demands of her job. Since adolescence she has suffered from depression, for which she is currently being treated. She has a high school diploma, and has pursued an interest in animal care through employment as a veterinarian assistant and a pet sitter/groomer. She is employed part-time due to the fact that she tires easily. She spends her free time socializing with friends and pursuing several interests, including skydiving, at which she is quite adept. She functions fairly independently in that she drives a car and lives by herself in an apartment. However, her parents pay her rent and some of her living expenses. Shortly after her assessment, J. moved across the country to live with her boyfriend (and find employment).

## Case Study 2

D. is a 21-year-old male with a full scale IQ of 76 (verbal IQ, 79; performance IQ, 77). His adaptive living skills are commensurate with his IQ, although he also has difficulties in expressive language skills and in the management of his own money. He was treated for ADHD during childhood, but does not display any psychiatric symptoms at this time. He has a high school diploma and has worked part-time for the past three years as an usher at a local movie theater. He spends his free time socializing with friends and playing video games. He does not drive a car, and relies on public transportation or rides from family. He lives at home with his parents and does not have plans to live independently at this time.

Educators working with children with a neurocognitive impairment will need to do assessments to identify areas of strengths and weaknesses. Only then can a specially tailored education program best benefit the child. In the specific case of a child with VCFS, many different domains should be explored.

## LEARNING ISSUES

Learning issues associated with VCFS include:

- Difficulty with problem solving, abstract reasoning, or making inferences
- Poor executive function (ability to approach a new problem, solve it, and evaluate the performance; reasoning)

- Difficulty with initiative and self regulation
- Problems with remembering multistep directions or complex verbal information (slow processing speed and inefficient mental flexibility)
- Deficits in attention (on task behavior and concentration)
- Problems with initial encoding of information (remembering new vocabulary, recalling information)
- Depressed working memory (ability to hold information in mind long enough to perform complex tasks)
- Easily frustrated and distractible
- Trouble with math problem solving and understanding the logic behind math concepts (inductive and deductive reasoning skills)
- Weak reading comprehension skills (drawing conclusions, using context clues, recognizing cause and effect, making inferences)
- Difficulty elaborating on thoughts in written form
- Low crystallized knowledge (language development, lexical knowledge, listening ability, general information, and information about culture)
- Poor organization of information (synthesis, analysis, sequencing)
- Poor communication ability (ability to speak in "real life" situations in a manner that transmits ideas, thoughts, or feelings)
- Weak receptive language skills (ability to follow simple instructions)
- Difficulty with visual reasoning (ability to do visual problem-solving tasks, awareness of visual details, visual perception, and judgment of lines and angles)
- Trouble with visual processing (ability to generate, perceive, analyze, store, and manipulate visual patterns and stimuli—spatial relations, visual memory, closure speed, visualization, form constancy, spatial scanning)
- Difficulty with large group presentations, note taking, or gaining information from videos
- Variable test taking skills: will likely not generalize knowledge to novel situations, may not understand format of test, may make careless errors, may not be able to express knowledge in essay format, may tire easily, may not be able to recall learned information without cues, uneven test performance
- Various behavior challenges (attention deficit disorder, mood swings, internalizing problems, occasionally disruptive, impulsive, separation anxiety)

■ Poor adaptive skills (needed for independent living)

Many VCFS children do show relative areas of strengths. These include:

■ Rote math calculations using given formulas

■ Reading, decoding, and understanding basic information

■ Rote memory (especially for lists)

■ Ability to remember well-encoded information

■ Spelling and grammar

■ Simple focused attention

■ Computer skills

■ Word processing speed

■ Kinesthetic abilities (such as learning dance or karate)

■ Rhythm and musical talent

■ Willingness to learn

■ Pleasant personality

Many VCFS students can progress through a typical school curriculum at a slower pace and with modifications. Others will need more intense instruction in a smaller, more structured setting. Many do best in a small class format for at least part of the day.

The majority of VCFS students learn to read, do basic math, and understand a general social studies and science curriculum. It is interesting to note that many reportedly excel in music, so this area may offer a positive outlet for a student who will likely have challenges with the regular academic curriculum. Some VCFS young adults have been quite successful in musical performance and a few have pursued teaching careers. Some have completed post-secondary degrees, married, and lead typical lives. Others pursue less academic outlets and hold jobs in a nonprofessional sector such as in service or retail. A large number of adults, however, need assistance with independent living skills, work on only a part-time basis, and get help from their family or from the government. As mentioned earlier, a substantial number also are plagued with psychiatric issues that interfere with leading a productive adult life.

Once a diagnosis of VCFS is made, all children should be given an age-appropriate neurocognitive evaluation. This should include an assessment of:

■ Cognitive ability

■ Academic achievement

■ Problem-solving/reasoning ability

■ Auditory processing

■ Fine/gross motor skills

■ Memory (visual and auditory)

■ Processing speed

■ Visual/spatial ability

■ Language skills (expressive and receptive)

■ Behavior

■ Social skills

■ Life skills

## TESTING CONSIDERATIONS

There are numerous tests on the market that can assess these domains. Most of these tests can be found at the following Web sites: http://www.psych-ed publications.com, http://www.schoolpsychology.net, or http://www.psych test.com. They can also be purchased through the publishing companies listed below. An additional Web site that is helpful for reviews of psychological tests is http://www.buros.unl.edu.

Some of the more commonly used assessment tools are the following.

Tests of general cognitive ability:

1. For infants through age 2.5: Bayley Scales of Infant Development, 2nd or 3rd edition (BSID-II) (N. Bayley), PsychCorp-Harcourt Assessment Inc., http://www.psychcorp.com

2. For preschoolers: Stanford-Binet Intelligence Scale, 4th edition; Wechsler Preschool and Primary Scale of Intelligence (WPPSI), 3rd edition (D. Wechsler), PsychCorp-Harcourt Assessment Inc., http://www.psychcorp.com

3. For school-aged children: Wechsler Intelligence Scale for Children, 4th edition (WISC-IV) (D. Wechsler et al.), PsychCorp-Harcourt Assessment Inc., http://www.psychcorp.com

4. Kaufman Assessment Battery for Children, 2nd edition (KABC-II) (A. Kaufman and L. Kaufman), AGS Publishing Co, http://www.agsnet.com

Tests of achievement:

1. Wechsler Individual Achievement Test, 2nd edition (WIAT-II) (D. Wechsler), PsychCorp-Harcourt Assessment Inc., http://www.psychcorp.com

2. Woodcock Johnson Test of Achievement III (R. Woodcock, K. McGrew, and N. Mather), http://www.riverpub.com

Tests of problem solving:

1. Wisconsin Card Sorting Task (R. Heaton et al.), Psychological Assessment Resources, http://www.parinc.com

2. Test of Problem Solving (TOPS), Lingui Systems Inc., East Moline, IL

3. NEPSY A Developmental Neuropsychological Assessment (M. Korman, U. Kirk, and S. Kemp), PsychCorp-Harcourt Assessment Inc., http://www.psychcorp.com

Tests of visual perception:

1. Beery-Buktenica Developmental Test of Visual-Motor Integration (VMI), (K. Beery and N. Buktenica), Modern Curriculum Press, Columbus, Ohio

2. Rey-Osterrieth Complex Figure Test (J. Meyers and K. Meyer), Psychological Assessment Resources, http://www.parinc.com

Tests of behavior:

1. Behavior Assessment System for Children (BASC), American Guidance Service, Inc., http://www.agsnet.com

2. C. Connors Rating Scales Revised (CRS-R) (C. Connors, Keith, J. Epstein, and D. Johnson), Multi-Health Systems, Inc., http://www.mhs.com

3. School Social Behavior Scales (SSBS) (K. Merrell), http://www.assessmentintervention.com

4. Child Behavior Checklist (CBCL) (T. Achenbach, 1998), http://www.aseba.org

5. Achenbach System of Empirically Based Assessment (T. Achebach et al, 2005), http://www.aseba.org

Tests of attention:

1. Connors Continuous Performance Test-II (CPT), Multi-Health Systems, Inc., http://www.mhs.com

Tests of life/social skills:

1. Vineland Adaptive Behavior Scales (VABS) (S. Sparrow, D. Balla, D. Cicchetti, and P. Harrison), American Guidance Service, http://www.agsnet.com

2. Functional Assessment and Intervention System-Improving School Behavior (FAIS) (K. Stoiber), PsychCorp-Harcourt Assessment Inc., http://www.psychcorp.com

3. Social Skills Rating Scales (SSRS) (F. Gresham and S. Elliot), American Guidance Service Publishing, http://www.agsnet.com

4. Scales of Independent Behavior-Revised (SIB-R) (R. Bruininks, R. Woodcock, R. Weatherman, and B. Hill), Riverside Publishing, http://www.riverpub.com

5. Autism Diagnostic Interview-Revised (ADI-R) (C. Lord, M. Rutter, and A. LeCouteur, 1994), Western Psychological Services, http://www.wpspublish.com

6. Autism Diagnostic Observation Schedule (ADOS) (C. Lord, M. Rutter, A. DiLavore, and Risi, 1999), Western Psychological Services, http://www.wpspublish.com

7. Adaptive Behavior Assessment System (ABAS) (P. Harrison and T. Oakland), PsychCorp-Harcourt Assessment Inc., http://www.psychcorp.com

Tests of speech and language:

1. NEPSY (Language and Memory), PsychCorp-Harcourt Assessment Inc., http://www.psychcorp.com

2. California Verbal Learning Test (CVLT) (D. Delis, J. Kramer, E. Kaplan, B. Ober, and A. Fridlund), PsychCorp-Harcourt Assessment Inc., http://www.psychcorp.com

3. Conversational speech samples

4. Test of Written Language-III (TOWL) (D. Hammill and S. Larson), Pro-Ed Publisher, http://www.proedinc.com

5. Test of Pragmatic Language (TOPL) (D. Phelps-Terasaki and T. Phelps-Gunn), Pro-Ed Publisher, http://www.proedinc.com

6. Test of Language Development (TOLD) (D. Hammill and P. Newcomer), Pro-Ed Publisher, http://www.proedinc.com

7. Clinical Evaluation of Language Fundamentals (CELF) (E. Semel, E. Wilg, and W. Secord), PsychCorp-Harcourt Assessment Inc., http://www.psychcorp.com

There is one point that should be carefully considered when testing is used for school placement. IQ testing is not necessarily an accurate predictor of school performance in this population. Some typically used IQ tests are timed, which puts a child with low muscle tone and slowed processing speed at a distinct disadvantage. Children with VCFS are very poor test takers and their performance is highly variable. They are anxious, give up easily, and may be inattentive or impulsive. A low IQ score is not necessarily predictive of learning ability and should *never* be used as the sole reason to place a VCFS child in a restrictive classroom with severely impaired peers. The vast majority of VCFS students are more appropriately placed in the regular mainstream education program with support from the special education team.

Children with VCFS also need to be assessed carefully in the areas of behavior and adaptive skills. Activities of daily living and acquiring life skills are many times at a lower level than one would expect. These children should also be screened for behavioral difficulties multiple times during their school-age years. As stated earlier, it is relatively common for VCFS children to develop psychological difficulties as they mature. It is therefore imperative that these issues are addressed in any educational program.

Several studies have indicated that many VCFS children meet the criteria of a nonverbal learning disability. The common characteristics of a nonverbal learning disability are as follows (Thompson, 1997; Rourke, 1989).

- Performance IQ significantly lower than verbal IQ (spread of more than 10 points)

- Excellent spelling skills, early reading skills

- Attention to details, but not to the "whole" or *gestalt*

- Gross and fine motor difficulties

- Visual and/or auditory memory problems

- Difficulty keeping track of things

- Difficulties with concept formation, including generation of strategies, problem solving, abstract reasoning

- Trouble with spatial problems

- Difficulty following through with assignments without close supervision

- Difficulty sustaining attention except when interested in tasks

- Difficulty initiating activities on own (e.g., beginning homework assignments on own)

- Impulsive behavior

- Poor social judgment (misreads social cues, body language, etc.)

- Appears unmotivated

- Seeks more assistance in doing daily living skills than is actually required

- Difficulty naming or defining things

- Difficulty copying things from the board

When one compares the typical findings of the VCFS profile, there are many similarities between this learning profile and a child with nonverbal learning disabilities. Even without the performance and verbal IQ discrepancies often seen with a nonverbal learning disability (NVLD), most VCFS students will encounter many of the same learning obstacles. However, the VCFS student's challenges are usually harder to overcome because of the added language difficulties, attention issues, chronic health problems, lower cognitive ability, and compounding psychiatric diagnoses. Therefore, although many accommodations recommended for use with NVLD students can also be applied to VCFS youngsters, accommodations should not be limited to those recommended for NVLD children since the disabilities of VCFS children go beyond NVLD.

A comprehensive list of suggested accommodations can be found in the appendix and throughout the book.

The following is a timeline for education-related interventions.

Birth to 3:

- Evaluation by speech and language professionals, occupational therapists, and physical therapists

- Possible interventions include speech therapy, with emphasis on intelligibility and language fundamentals, occupational therapy to improve fine motor skills, hypotonia, and balance, and physical therapy to strengthen gross motor skills

Ages 3 to 5:

- Continued speech therapy, occupational therapy (OT), and physical therapy if needed

- Intensive math readiness instruction

- Phonemic awareness instruction

- Preschool to learn pre-reading skills, social interaction skills, and listening skills and to foster independence

- Play group to reinforce communication with others and to learn appropriate social behavior

- Other possible options for developing skills—early music opportunities (e.g., Suzuki, Yamaha music, etc.), gymnastics, karate, soccer, etc.

Ages 5 to 8:

- Evaluation for school assistance through special education

- Continued speech, OT, physical therapies if needed

- Additional instruction in math and reading including after school/ home involvement

- Therapy to improve memory, attention, and cognition

- Home/school program to teach independence skills

- Social skills instruction

Ages 9 to 11:

- Comprehensive reevaluation, including IQ testing, prior to entry to middle school

- Continued support through special education at school

- Continued therapy, if necessary

- Continued additional interventions in math and reading

- Direct instruction in organization skills, test taking, school success strategies

- Participation in a friendship group or other organized activity

- Social skills training; ideally, this should be provided through the school system, with a focus on social interaction and language pragmatics; social skills training could also be provided by either mental health professionals or speech-language specialists

- Continued training and monitoring of independent living skills

- Optional involvement in after school activities such as sports, music, dance, etc.

Ages 12 to 15:

- Comprehensive reevaluation, including IQ testing, prior to entry to high school

- Continued support through special education

- More intensive assistance with study skills

- One-on-one tutoring assistance with academic subjects

- Continued after school remediation in math and reading

- Direct training in memory techniques

- Career exploration and job shadowing opportunities

- Continued direct instruction with social skills

- Continued independent living skills training

- Consider away from home experience for a short time period (camp, travel)
- Optional involvement in after school activities

Ages 16 to 18:

- Continued support through special education
- One-on-one tutoring assistance
- Vocational assessment to determine possible job placements
- Work experience opportunities
- College/post-secondary explorations and planning
- Life skills assessment and independent living skills training
- Possible driving training
- Direct instruction in sex education and legal issues associated with adulthood
- Direct assistance with connecting family to community-based supports for adults with special needs
- Social skills training if needed
- Opportunities to participate in clubs, sports, music groups, etc.

Ages 18 to 21:

- Placement in a college program, technical school, or work apprenticeship program
- Additional training in independent living skills
- One-on-one tutoring assistance
- Job coaching in a work environment
- Possible away from home living opportunity in a dorm, apartment, etc., with assistance
- Continued social skills assistance if needed
- Assistance with applying for community support

**Acknowledgments:** Information on the cognitve profile of children with VCFS was in part derived from T. J. Simon, M. Burg, & D. Gothelf.. (2007). Cognitive and behavioral characteristics of children with chromosome 22q11.2 deletion. In M. M. M. Mazzocco & J. L. Ross (Eds.), *Neurogenetic Developmental Disorders: Manifestation and Identification in Childhood.* Cambridge, MA: MIT Press.

# REFERENCES

Antshel, K., AbdulSabur., N, Higgins, A. M., Shprintzen, R. J., & Kates, W. R. (2006). Neuropsychological and community functioning in adults with velocardiofacial syndrome. Unpublished.

Antshel, K., AbdulSabur, N., Roizen, N., Fremont, W., & Kates, W. R. (2005). Sex differences in cognitive functioning in velocardiofacial syndrome (VCFS). *Developmental Neuropsychology*, *28*(3), 849–869.

Bayley, N. (1969). *Bayley scales of infant development*. New York: Psychological Corporation.

Bearden, C. E., Jawed, A. F., Lynch, D. R., Monterosso J. R., Sokol, S., McDonald-McGinn, D. M., et al. (2005). Effects of COMT genotype on behavioral symptomatology in the 22q11.2 deletion syndrome. *Child Neuropsychology*, *11*(1), 109–117.

Bearden, C. E., Woodin, M. F., Wang, P. P., Moss, E., McDonald-McGinn, D., Zachai, E., et al. (2001). The neurocognitive phenotype of the 22q11.2 deletion syndrome: Selective deficit in visual-spatial memory. *Journal of Clinical and Experimental Neuropsychology*, *23*(4), 447–464.

Campbell, L., & Swillen, A. (2005). The cognitive spectrum in velo-cardio-facial syndrome. In K. C. Murphy & P. J. Scramble (Eds.), *Velo-Cardio-Facial Syndrome: A Model for Understanding Microdeletion Disorders* (pp.147–164). Cambridge, UK: Cambridge University Press.

De Smedt, B., Swillen, A., Devriendt, K., Fryns, J. P., Verschaffel, L., & Ghesquiere, P. (2007). Mathematical disabilities in children with velo-cardio-facial syndrome. *Neuropsychologia*, *45*, 885–895.

Fine, S., Weissman, A., Gerdes, M., Pinto-Martin, J., Zackai, E., McDonald-McGinn, D., et. al. (2005). Autism spectrum disorders and symptoms in children with molecularly confirmed 22q11.2 deletion syndrome. *Journal of Autism and Developmental Disorders*, *35*(4), 461–470.

Gerdes, M., Solot, C., Wang, P. P., McDonald-McGinn, D. M., & Zackai, E. H. (2001). Taking advantage of early diagnosis: Preschool children with the 22q11.2 deletion. *Genetics in Medicine*, *3*(1), 40–44.

Gerdes, M., Solot, C., Wang, P. P., Moss, E. M., LaRossa, D., Randall, P., et al. (1999). Cognitive and behavior profile of preschool children with chromosome 22q11.2 deletion. *American Journal of Medical Genetics*, *85*, 127–133.

Glaser, B., Mumme, D. L., Blasey, C., Morris, M. A., Dahoun, S. P., Antonarakis, S. E., et al. (2002). Language skills in children with velocardiofacial syndrome (deletion 22q11.2). *The Journal of Pediatrics*, *140*, 753–758.

Golding-Kushner, K., Weller, G., & Shprintzen, R. J. (1985). Velo-cardio-facial syndrome: Language and psychological profiles. *Journal of Craniofacial Genetics and Development Biology*, *5*, 259–266.

Gothelf, D. (2006, July). *Risk factors and developmental trajectories in VCFS*. Presentation at the 12th Annual International Scientific Meeting, Strasbourg, France.

Gothelf, D., Eliez, S., Thompson, T., Hinard, C., Penniman, L., Feinstein, C., et al. (2005). COMT genotype predicts longitudinal cognitive decline and psychosis in 22q11.2 deletion syndrome. *Nature Neuroscience*, *8*, 1500–1502.

Henry, J. C., van Amelsvoort, T., Morris, R. G., Owen, M. J., Murphy, D. G. M., & Murphy, K. C. (2002). An investigation of the neuropsychological profile in adults with velo-cardio-facial syndrome (VCFS). *Neuropsychologia*, *40*, 471–478.

Kates, W. (2006, July). *What can functional brain imaging tell us about cognition and emotion in VCFS?* Presentation at the 12th Annual International Scientific Meeting, Strasbourg, France.

Kok, L. L., & Solman, R. T. (1995). Velocardiofacial syndrome: Learning difficulties and intervention. *Journal of Medical Genetics, 32*(8), 612–618.

Korkman, M., Kirk, U., & Kemp, S. (1998). NEPSY: *A neurodevelopmental neuropsychological assessment.* San Antonio, TX: The Psychological Corporation.

Moss, E. M. (2001). Neuropsychological profile of children and adolescents with the 22q11.2 microdeletion. *Genetics in Medicine, 3*(1), 34–39.

Moss, E. M., Batshaw, M. L., Solot, C. B., Gerdes, M., Mcdonald-McGinn, D. M., Driscoll, D. A., et al. (1999). Psychoeducational profile of the 22q11.2 microdeletion: A complex pattern. *The Journal of Pediatrics, 134*(2), 193–198.

Niklasson, L., Rasmussen, P., Oskarsdottir, S., & Gillberg, C. (2002). Chromosome 22q11 deletion syndrome (CATCH 22), Neuropsychiatric and neuropsychological aspects. *Developmental Medicine and Child Neurology, 44*, 44–50.

Niklasson, L., Rasmussen, P., Oskarsdottir, S., & Gillberg, C. (2006, July). *Neuropsychiatric and behavioral problems in 100 individuals with 22q11 deletion syndrome.* Presentation at the 12th Annual International Scientific Meeting, Strasbourg, France.

Papolos, D. F., Faedda, G. L., Veit, S., Goldberg, R., Morrow, B., Kucherlapati, R., et al. (1996). Bipolar spectrum disorders in patients diagnosed with velo-cardio-facial syndrome: Does a hemizygous deletion of chromosome 22q11 result in bipolar affective disorder? *American Journal of Psychiatry, 153*(12), 1541–1547.

Rourke, B. (1989). *Nonverbal learning disabilities: The syndrome and the model.* New York: Guilford Press.

Scherer, N. J., D'Antonio, L. L., & Kalbfleisch, J. H. (1999). Early speech and language development in children with velocardiofacial syndrome. *American Journal of Medical Genetics, 88*(6) 714–723.

Shprintzen, R. J. (2000). Velo-cardio-facial syndrome: A distinct behavioral phenotype. *Mental Retardation and Developmental Disability Research Reviews, 6*, 142–147.

Sobin, C., Kiley-Brabeck, K., Daniels, S., Khuri, J., Taylor, L., Blundell, M., et al. (2005). Neuropsychological characteristics of children with the 22q11 deletion syndrome: A descriptive analysis. *Child Neuropsychology, 11*(1), 39–53.

Solot, C. B., Gerdes, M., Kirschner, R. E., McDonald-McGinn, D. M., Moss, E., Woodin, M., et al. (2001). Communication issues in 22q11.2 deletion syndrome: Children at risk. *Genetics in Medicine, 3*(1), 67–71.

Sparrow, S. S., Balla, D. A., & Cichetti, D. V. (1984). Vineland Adaptive Behavior Scales (Interview ed.). Circle Pines, MN: American Guidance Service.

Swillen, A., Devriendt, K., & Legius, E. (1999). The behavioral phenotype in velo-cardio-facial syndrome (VCFS). *Genetic Counseling, 10*(1), 79–88.

Swillen A. (2006, July). *Longitudinal data on intelligence in VCFS: From preschool to puberty.* Presentation at the 12th Annual International Scientific Meeting, Strasbourg, France.

Thompson, S. (1997). *The source for nonverbal learning disorders.* East Moline, IL: LinguiSystems.

Van Aken, K., Swillen, A., Gewillig, M., Devriendt, K., Van Roie, A., Simons, J., et al. (2006, July). *Motor development in children with a deletion 22q11 syndrome.* Presentation at the 12th Annual International Scientific Meeting, Strasbourg, France.

Vortsman, J., Morcus, M., Duiff, S., Klaassen, W. J., Heineman-de Boer, J., Beemer, F., et al. (2006). The 22q11.2 deletion in children: High rate of autistic disorders and early onset of psychotic symptoms. *Journal of the American Academy of Child and Adolescent Psychiatry*, *45*(9), 1104–1113.

Wang, P. P., Woodin, M. F., Kreps-Falk, R., & Moss, E. M. (2000). Research on behavioral phenotypes: Velocardiofacial syndrome (deletion 22q11.2). *Developmental Medicine & Child Neurology*, *42*, 422–427.

Wechsler, D. (1991). Wechsler Intelligence Scale for Children (3rd ed.). San Antonio, TX: Psychological Corporation.

Wechsler, D. (2001). Wechsler Individual Achievement Test (2nd ed.). San Antonio, TX: Psychological Corporation.

Woodin. M. F., Wang, P. P., Aleman, D., McDonald-McGinn, D. M., Zackai, E. H., & Moss, E. M. (2001). Neuropsychological profile of children and adolescents with the 22q11.2 microdeletion. *Genetics in Medicine*, *3*(1), 34–39.

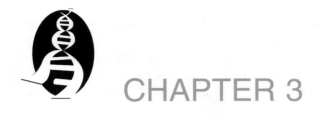

CHAPTER 3

# Cognition and the VCFS Brain

## *The Implications of Syndrome-Specific Deficits for School Performance*

BRONWYN GLASER, MA and STEPHAN ELIEZ, MD

## WHAT CAN A DIAGNOSIS OF VCFS TELL US ABOUT ACADEMIC PERFORMANCE?

Although many of the exact mechanisms linking brain changes to learning problems remain to be discovered, consideration of what is known thus far can provide information useful in planning the education of a child affected by a microdeletion 22q11 (22q11DS). This chapter focuses on the cognitive difficulties that are most consistently demonstrated in the syndrome and likely to present significant challenges to the learning of a child with VCFS. In the chapter sections, we describe and discuss related brain changes for the following difficulties: attention problems, mathematics reasoning, visuo-spatial reasoning, face and object processing, and motor problems. Our principal goal was to provide useful summaries of the impairments and underlying neuroanatomy for practitioners who do not necessarily have backgrounds in neuroscience. For this reason, at times we simplify in order to present the information as clearly as possible. No region of the brain works in isolation; and although we sometimes focus on one particular region to illustrate a point, it is important to mention that the circuitry in each of the discussed impairments is complex and integrative.

Commonly noted speech and language impairments in VCFS (Glaser et al., 2002; Golding-Kushner, Weller, & Shprintzen, 1985; Scherer D'Antonio, & Kalbfleisch, 1999; Solot et al., 2001; Solot et al., 2000) are the subject of a separate chapter in this volume (see Chapter 5) and therefore are not discussed here. There is evidence of key developmental changes to language delays in the syndrome; with pronounced early deficits in comprehension and production (Gerdes et al., 1999; Golding-Kushner et al., 1985; Scherer et al., 1999), mixed evidence for gains in production at school age, due perhaps in part to speech therapy and surgical interventions (Glaser et al., 2002; Solot et al., 2000), and subsequent decline in adolescence (Gothelf et al., 2005). The unique speech and language issues associated with VCFS require frequent monitoring and evaluations, and thus a separate chapter has been devoted to the subject.

## WHY DO CHILDREN WITH VCFS HAVE LOWER IQ SCORES?

Children and adolescents affected by 22q11DS suffer from learning disabilities and mild to moderate mental retardation (Swillen et al., 1997), with total IQ scores of 70–80 relative to an average score of 100 (Moss et al., 1999; Swillen et al., 1999; van Amelsvoort, Henry, et al., 2004). On average, nonverbal or performance IQ is generally lower than verbal IQ (Moss et al., 1999; Swillen et al., 1999; Woodin et al., 2001); just as visual memory, and especially visuo-spatial memory, is frequently more impaired than verbal memory (Bearden et al., 2001; Woodin et al., 2001). Associated memory impairments likely affect cognitive performance and learning difficulties in the syndrome and are discussed along with the specific impairments in this chapter.

Brain imaging studies have consistently shown that children with VCFS have smaller overall brains consisting of less gray (neurons) and white matter (the bundles of axons connecting neurons) (Figure 3–1) than typically developing children. Abnormal brain development, resulting in changes to gray matter volumes, often corresponds to reductions in IQ (Reiss, Abrams, Singer, Ross, & Denckla, 1996; Wilke, Sohn, Byars, & Holland, 2003), which may partially explain the occurrence of mental retardation in the syndrome. Although no region of the brain works in isolation, many of the following sections describe learning difficulties that are at least partially linked to changes in the parietal lobe (Figure 3–2), a region that is particularly reduced in the VCFS brain. Previous studies on brain changes in VCFS have consistently shown parietal gray matter to be reduced above and beyond reductions affecting the whole brain (Zinkstok & van Amelsvoort, 2005). Moreover, white matter is reduced, suggesting decreased connectivity between lobes as well as within the parietal lobe (Barnea-Goraly et al., 2003; T. J. Simon, Ding, et al., 2005). Finally, changes to cortical folding were recently demonstrated in VCFS, with fewer surface folds especially apparent in the frontal and parietal lobes

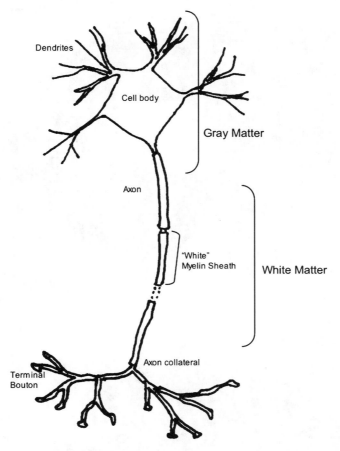

**FIGURE 3–1.** This schematic drawing of a neuron shows the cell bodies and myelinated axons comprising gray and white matter.

(Schaer et al., 2005). These changes to the structure of the brain especially suggest abnormal wiring, and thus abnormal function, in the parietal lobe (Figure 3-2).

## ARE ATTENTION PROBLEMS COMMON IN VCFS?

Attention problems are among the most frequent behavioral observations in the syndrome and likely impact an affected child's performance in most other cognitive domains. Indeed, most studies measuring psychopathology associated with the disorder have demonstrated that 30–50% of individuals affected

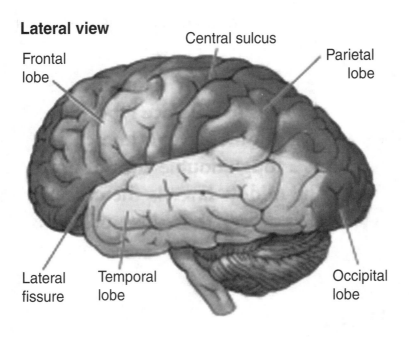

**Lateral view**

Frontal lobe

Central sulcus

Parietal lobe

Lateral fissure

Temporal lobe

Occipital lobe

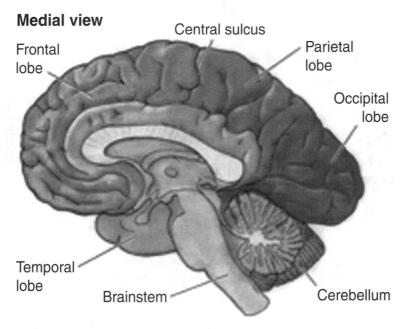

**Medial view**

Frontal lobe

Central sulcus

Parietal lobe

Occipital lobe

Temporal lobe

Brainstem

Cerebellum

**FIGURE 3–2.** The major lobes and divisions of the brain. (Reprinted with permission from An "Introduction to Brain and Behavior", by B. Kolb and I. Q. Whislaw, p. 42. Copyright 2001 Worth Publishers.)

by VCFS meet criteria for ADHD (Baker & Skuse, 2005; Feinstein et al., 2002; Gothelf et al., 2004; Niklasson Rasmussen, Oskarsdottir, & Gillberg, 2001). In addition to high rates of ADHD diagnoses, we have observed that children and adolescents with VCFS often exhibit especially high rates of inattentive-type symptoms; posing a challenge to tasks such as focusing in class, keeping up with lessons, and organizing assignments and belongings. Although it is unclear whether attention problems are secondary to the lower than average IQ in VCFS (Baker & Skuse, 2005; Feinstein, Eliez, Blasey, & Reiss, 2002), or whether VCFS may share a genetic basis with ADHD pathologies (Bish. Ferrante, McDonald-McGinn, Zackai, & Simon, 2005), the high rates of attention problems become an important consideration in a school environment.

Cognitive studies have searched for evidence of attention problems in affected individuals' treatment of information. Focusing on an ability to organize information, as well as the ability to disregard distracting irrelevant information, appears to be at the core of our ability to concentrate on a stimulus (Posner & Petersen, 1990). Children with VCFS, compared to normal children, demonstrate a larger than usual effect from the presence of distracter information during an attention task (Bish et al., 2005; Sobin et al., 2004). Moreover, the presence of distracters continues to hurt their performance, whereas normal children are better at overcoming this influence. These difficulties in executive control likely affect most academic tasks involving the processing and interpretation of information and the application of previous learning. Indeed, impairments in abilities involving the processing and organization of information known as executive functions, and including abilities such as working memory (the ability to keep information in one's mind while performing a transformation with it), set shifting (the cognitive flexibility needed to change the set of rules one applies to a task), and planning (the ability to anticipate necessary adjustments to complete a task), are thought to underlie many of the cognitive deficits and memory impairments observed in VCFS (Sobin et al., 2004; Wang, Woodin, Kreps-Falk & Moss, 2000; Woodin et al., 2001).

Attention problems are rarely discussed without mention of disruptions to the networks linking the frontal lobe and the corpus striatum, a component of the basal ganglia that is located inward from the outer cortex (Figure 3–3). Frontal-striatal networks, involving the dorsolateral prefrontal cortex, the caudate, the putamen, and the globus pallidus, are thought to be especially important to the control of posture and movement (Seidman, Valera, & Makris, 2005). The volume of the caudate in particular has been related to the planning of self-generated novel action (Monchi, Petrides, Strafella, Worsley, & Doyon, 2006). Disorders of movement control, such as Parkinson's disease, Huntington's disease, and ADHD have all been considered in light of impairments in the regulation of dopamine, and related neurotransmitters, in frontal-striatal connections.

Reductions in the frontal lobe, and the dorsolateral prefrontal cortex in particular (Kates et al., 2005), as well as increased caudate volumes (Eliez, Barnea-Goraly, Schmitt, Liu & Reiss, 2002), provide evidence for frontal-striatal

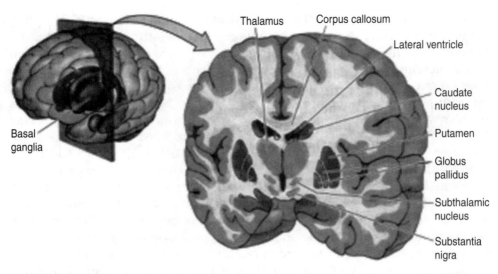

**FIGURE 3–3.** The structures of the basal ganglia, which are discussed in the context of attention and motor problems. (Reprinted with permission from "An Introduction to Brain and Behavior", by B. Kolb and I. Q. Whislaw, p. 58. Copyright 2001 Worth Publishers.)

impairments in VCFS. Further, medications such as methylphenidate, which increase synaptic catecholamines, and especially dopamine, in frontal-striatal circuits, have been shown to positively impact attention problems in ADHD as well as VCFS (Gothelf et al., 2003). Alterations to the corpus callosum (Shashi et al., 2004; T. J. Simon, Ding, et al., 2005) (Figure 3–2), which contributes to connectivity between the two hemispheres of the brain especially in the frontal and cerebellar regions, and the cerebellum (Figure 3–2), traditionally known for its involvement in motor functions but also known to play a significant role in cognitive learning and behavioral changes (Schmahmann, 2004), have been consistently reported in ADHD (Seidman et al., 2005) and VCFS (Eliez, Schmitt, et al., 2001; van Amelsvoort, Daly, et al., 2004; van Amelsvoort, Daly, et al., 2001; Zinkstok & van Amelsvoort, 2005). These neuroanatomical similarities suggest that the neurobiology underlying attention problems in ADHD and VCFS may be similar.

In addition to evidence for similar structural impairments, shifts and disengagement of attention from a stimulus are related to neuronal activity in the superior parietal lobe and have recently been related to posterior parietal lobe reductions in VCFS (T. J. Simon, Bearden, et al., 2005). An inability to disengage from a stimulus is backed by regional reductions in the frontal and parietal lobes (Figure 3–2), as well as reduced connectivity between the two regions (Barnea-Goraly et al., 2003; T. J. Simon, Ding, et al., 2005). In summary, the structural changes observed in VCFS give us multiple reasons to expect problems in attention and executive control among affected individuals.

# WHY IS MATH PARTICULARLY DIFFICULT FOR MOST AFFECTED CHILDREN?

Mathematics deficiencies are one of the most primordial and consistently observed cognitive weaknesses associated with VCFS. Mathematics impairments were singled out early in papers first describing the cognitive profile of the syndrome (Golding-Kushner et al., 1985; Kok & Solman, 1995; Swillen et al., 1997). Several studies have documented how difficult it is for an affected child to learn rote mathematical facts or retain mathematical concepts (Moss et al., 1999; Swillen et al., 1999; Wang et al., 2000; Woodin et al., 2001). Parents continually worry about their child's difficulty to learn basic math skills, and affected children readily admit how much they hate doing math mostly because they feel it is especially difficult for them. Moreover, math appears to be consistently deficient in children with VCFS despite their general level of functioning (Golding-Kushner et al., 1985).

Children with VCFS appear to be impaired on all types of mathematics from early on (De Smedt, Swillen, Ghesquiere, Devriendt, & Fryns, 2003). Swillen et al. reported delays in grade-level mental calculation and number system knowledge (both calculation and applied math) compared to reading and spelling tests (Swillen et al., 1999). Similarly, at least two studies found both rote math and math reasoning to be impaired on a math achievement test (Moss et al., 1999; Woodin et al., 2001). Although most affected children learn to count, we have observed that complex operations such as counting by multiples greater than 2 can pose a challenge. However, despite these difficulties, affected individuals remain capable of acquiring a basic level of math. A study solely devoted to investigating math in a group of adolescents with VCFS tracked accuracy on 2- and 3-operand arithmetic problems. Affected individuals appear to solve simple equations (2-operand) at rates comparable to controls, while experiencing more difficulty on complex equations (3-operand) relative to an age- and gender-matched control group (Eliez, Blasey, Schmitt, et al., 2001).

A difficulty solving complex equations, such as $4 + 5 - 2$, may represent additional difficulties with constructs other than numerical reasoning. Besides correctly perceiving the values of the numbers, a person solving the above equation must attend to the important information, use working memory skills to retain key information while performing the required math transformation, and self-monitor to verify the accuracy of the answer. Thus, a delay in the development of working memory likely perpetuates difficulties with complex math reasoning among affected individuals (De Smedt, Ghesquiere, & Swillen, 2005; Wang et al., 2000; Woodin et al., 2001). Children with VCFS have demonstrated difficulties manipulating information, or transforming the order of information, despite intact retention abilities (Majerus, Glaser, Van der Linden, & Eliez, 2006). This finding is concordant with aforementioned studies pointing to problems in executive control (Bish et al., 2005; Sobin et al.,

2004). Although their problems with math are likely compounded by difficulties acquiring and encoding numerical information due to alterations in parietal brain structure (see following paragraph), a weakness in executive control and manipulation of information certainly exacerbates this vulnerability.

Problems doing math are likely due to early and frequent structural changes to the posterior part of the brain. Indeed, numerical deficits in the syndrome have been specifically related to posterior parietal lobe reductions in the syndrome (T. J. Simon, Bearden, et al., 2005), and likely involve reductions in connectivity in areas around the intraparietal sulcus in particular (Barnea-Goraly, Eliez, Menon, Bammer, & Reiss, 2005) (Figure 3–4), a subregion frequently associated with mathematics. Alterations to connectivity in the parietal lobe also are supported by the aforementioned study investigating performance on simple and complex equations. Specifically, the localization of brain activity was recorded, in addition to accuracy, while the participants solved equations (Eliez, Blasey, Menon, et al., 2001). In addition to frontal lobe involvement and consistent with evidence for changes in regional connectivity (Barnea-Goraly et al., 2003), adolescents with VCFS showed increased activity in a subregion of the left side of the parietal lobe, called the supramarginal gyrus, located adjacent to the intraparietal sulcus (Eliez, Blasey, Menon, et al., 2001) (Figure 3–4). In summary, the neuroanatomical evidence indicates that changes to the parietal lobes likely contribute to the difficulty that

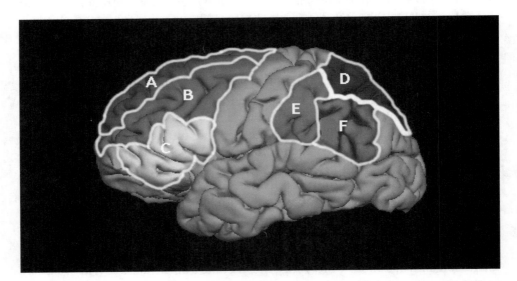

**FIGURE 3–4.** This picture of the brain illustrates key frontal and parietal regions. Superior frontal **(A)**, middle frontal **(B)**, and inferior frontal **(C)** divide the frontal lobes. The parietal lobes are divided into superior parietal **(D)**, supramarginal **(E)** and angular **(F)** gyri. The intraparietal sulcus, between the parietal sub-regions, is traced in white. Adapted from "Functional Brain Imaging Study of Mathematical Reasoning Abilities in Velocardiofacial Syndrome (del22q11.2)," by S. Eliez, C. M. Blasey, V. Menon, C. D. White, J. F. Schmitt, and A. L. Reiss, 2001, *Genetic Medicine, 3,* pp. 49–55.

individuals experience during complex math equations. Moreover, increased activation in the VCFS group suggests an increase in energy and lack of efficiency in the processing, which may render the coordination of numerical knowledge and problem-solving skills difficult for affected individuals.

## TO WHAT EXTENT IS VISUO-SPATIAL REASONING IMPAIRED IN VCFS?

The fact that spatial impairments are correlated with math performance in children with VCFS (Wang et al., 2000) and are associated with the parietal lobe (O. Simon et al., 2004) indicates that difficulties in visuo-spatial perception may be related to arithmetic impairments. Thus, to further define numerical deficits in the syndrome, it is important to concurrently consider visuo-spatial difficulties. Research points to a fundamental relationship between arithmetic and visuo-spatial deficits (Hubbard, Piazza, Pinel, & Dehaene, 2005). Indeed, numerical and visuo-spatial reasoning are inextricably linked in the function of a typical mature human brain. Investigations of numerical and visuo-spatial deficits show that we often think about numbers in terms of space, and that our conception and viewing of space greatly affects our conception of numbers (Hubbard et al., 2005). Although we first memorize mathematics facts as children, they quickly become automated and reinforced through visuo-spatial representations (e.g., a mental image representing the quantity of days and weeks in the yearly calendar); hence, it is not surprising that mathematical deficits frequently accompany problems in visuo-spatial reasoning.

Indeed, there is evidence showing that both judgments of numeracy and distance are less automated in children with VCFS. First of all, affected children appear to have more difficulties judging quantities than typically developing children. Using an enumeration task, where children were asked to identify the number of objects on display, Simon and colleagues found that children affected by the syndrome made more errors when counting objects and were slower to judge the number of objects displayed, particularly when the number could not be automatically estimated (T. J. Simon, Bearden, et al., 2005; T. J. Simon, Bish, et al., 2005). Moreover, the range of estimation for a child with VCFS tends to be more restricted than for a typically developing child, suggesting a weaker integration of counting numbers. Simon et al. further illustrated a difficulty connecting spatial and quantitative judgments through a distance task. Children with VCFS appeared to have more difficulty judging values of numbers clustered around a target number, such as 4 and 6 compared to 5. This "distance" effect represents an association between spatial and numerical deficits in the syndrome. The presence of a distance effect in VCFS also provides evidence for normal development in VCFS, since one would expect the capacities to be related in a normal brain.

Visuo-spatial impairments, independent of numerical difficulties, also have been reported in VCFS (Henry et al., 2002; Swillen et al., 1997). It has been proposed that children with VCFS are impaired on visuo-spatial short-term memory tasks (Bearden et al., 2001; Woodin et al., 2001), adding evidence for insufficient encoding and recall of visuo-spatial information compared to visual object recognition or verbal recall. The task shown to be deficient by Bearden et al. (2001) tests a child's ability to reproduce a pattern of dots on a grid after three separate exposures to the pattern. Further, using the same task, we have observed that even though children with VCFS improve their scores with repeated exposure to the pattern, the amount of learning, or improvement, is significantly less than with repeated exposure to words. However, the picture is complicated by the fact that children with VCFS do not always demonstrate a relative weakness on visuo-spatial memory tasks (Sobin et al., 2005), which may be due to changing task demands, the amount of material or working memory involved in the task, and time of exposure. In order to better understand the specific visuo-spatial memory problem in the syndrome, it will be important to try presenting different types of visuo-spatial material for more or less time to understand the circumstances that optimize acquisition. In addition to visuo-spatial memory, multiple components of visuo-spatial perception (form, angle, distance, and size reproduction abilities) need to be assessed to understand whether individuals perceive spatial stimuli in an accurate way.

Although the above cognitive evidence points to weakened parietal networks in VCFS, neuropsychological evaluations demonstrate that individuals are capable of learning both visuo-spatial and arithmetic skills. Thus, cerebral development in VCFS may be closer to normal than in other syndromes associated with more extreme cognitive difficulties. For example, Williams syndrome (WS) appears to be an extreme case of visuo-spatial and mathematics difficulties (Bellugi, Lichtenberger, Jones, Lai, & St. George, 2000) in that affected individuals start out with more severe impairments, which are compounded by abnormal development (Paterson, Girelli, Butterworth, & Karmiloff-Smith, 2006). The comparison between visuo-spatial skills in WS and VCFS is an excellent example of how a child's specific diagnosis can flag potential learning problems. Descriptions of associated deficits provide an initial road map, including indications for important divergences in development along the way. However, assumptions about an individual's functioning based solely on syndrome descriptions also can be harmful. Educational plans should always take a child's individual needs and functioning into account.

## DO CHILDREN WITH VCFS HAVE DIFFICULTIES WITH FACE AND OBJECT RECOGNITION?

The existence of visuo-spatial difficulties in VCFS opens the door to related questions. For example, could difficulties with visuo-spatial information be due to a general impairment in visual perception? If so, how do these impairments affect a child's perception of his surrounding visual world? Although researchers have yet to systematically investigate discrete components of object processing (i.e., recognition of form, color, detail, size, orientation) in VCFS, data point to stronger overall memory for objects than for locations (Bearden et al., 2001). However, despite evidence for stronger object memory, individuals with VCFS appear to have difficulties recognizing an object from its associated parts. Specifically, we have observed that affected individuals are slower than typically developing children at recognizing incomplete objects. Moreover, Henry et al. showed that adults with VCFS demonstrate difficulties recognizing objects from unusual viewpoints compared with IQ-matched developmentally delayed adults, further illustrating a deficit in the association of partial and complete pictures in developmentally mature individuals (Henry et al., 2002). These studies may suggest a tendency in the syndrome to treat visual objects partially, rather than in their entirety.

A similar observation has been made about face recognition in VCFS. We have observed that late in development, well into adolescence and early adulthood, children and adolescents with VCFS process faces by recognizing individual features rather than the ensemble. A 27-year-old adult female with the syndrome recently described this piecemeal strategy in the following way, "When given faces to remember, I look for differences in eyes, cheek definition, foreheads, and hair. It makes it easy to remember what one face looks like compared to another." Given the social nature of humans, as well as the importance that social interactions have on our ability to correctly perceive our environment, recognizing faces is vital. Although face processing does not reach adult levels until adolescence, young children begin processing faces and expressions early in infancy (Johnson, Dziurawiec, Ellis, & Morton, 1991). There is much evidence showing that as individuals become "experts" in processing and recognizing human faces and expressions, they perceive faces in an increasingly integrative way. In typically developing individuals, a piecemeal strategy is one of the first face processing strategies to develop and most young school-age children still show preferences for featural recognition of faces (Mondloch, Geldart, Maurer, & Le Grand, 2003). However, with maturity, we learn to process faces in their entirety, a strategy that becomes our preference by adolescence. Global processing has been called "quick and dirty" (Johnson, 2005) because it provides important immediate information about expressions and gaze, which give an emotional reading on social situations.

The neural mechanisms underlying face perception have recently received much attention in the field of cognitive neuroscience. In the following paragraphs, we apply some of the most recent findings to our results in VCFS. There is evidence for at least two concurrent cerebral routes for processing faces (Johnson, 2005). The first is a fast subcortical route linked to interpretation of information taken from the global composition of a face, such as gaze direction and emotional expression, and connecting to structures associated with social cognition, including the amygdala and the superior temporal sulcus (for reviews see Johnson, 2005, and Adolphs, 2003). A recent study illustrates the importance of the amygdala to emotion recognition by demonstrating a difficulty to recognize fearful expressions in a patient with amygdala damage (Adolphs, Tranel, & Buchanan, 2005). Thus, the biological drive to develop global processing likely accompanies maturity of emotion recognition and social development. A prominent delay in global processing, as seen in VCFS, may suggest a handicap in an affected individual's ability to read and react to emotions. Similar difficulties with face processing have been recorded for other neurogenetic conditions with social problems, such as autism, Williams syndrome, and schizophrenia.

A slower type of processing through a cortical route in temporal cortex, allowing for the recognition of facial characteristics and features (Vuilleumier, Armony, Driver, & Dolan, 2003), is associated with identifying and differentiating faces (Haxby, Hoffman, & Gobbini, 2000). This cortical route is part of the ventral visual processing pathway, which extends from the visual areas through the temporal lobe (Milner & Goodale, 1995; Mishkin & Ungerleider, 1982). Faces and categories of objects are recognized and differentiated by processing routes in temporal cortex (Haxby et al., 2001), all of which involve an area called the fusiform gyrus located at the inner juncture of the occipital and temporal lobes (Figure 3–2). The fusiform gyrus is most often discussed for its involvement in face processing (Kanwisher, McDermott, & Chun, 1997).

It may be that neuroanatomical changes to subcortical structures, such as the pulvinar in the thalamus (Bish, Nguyen, Ding, Ferrante, & Simon, 2004), as well as changes to axonal organization (Barnea-Goraly et al., 2005; Barnea-Goraly et al., 2003; T. J. Simon, Ding, et al., 2005), prevent normal development of the subcortical route and maturity of face processing skills in VCFS. This would explain why individuals with VCFS continue to use less efficient face processing strategies involving the fusiform gyrus and the ventral route, resulting in featural encoding and diminished social information. Further, although it appears to be the preferred strategy in VCFS, featural treatment of faces in affected individuals is still slower and less accurate than in typically developing individuals, pointing to possible structural changes to the fusiform gyrus and the ventral processing stream. This possibility is supported by an overall decrease in gray matter, suggesting specific regional reductions. The temporal lobe may be particularly susceptible to the effects of abnormal development as it is one of the slowest regions to reach mature levels of gray matter (Giedd et al., 1999). As a result, it is not surprising that previous neuroimaging studies suggest developmental alterations to the temporal lobe, with relatively preserved volumes reported in children and more decreased volumes reported in adults (Chow, Zipursky, Mikulis, & Bassett, 2002; Eliez, Blasey, Schmitt, et al., 2001; van Amelsvoort et al., 2001). This points to an increased risk for cognitive decline and aberrant development of object and face processing.

# HOW MIGHT MOTOR DELAYS BE RELATED TO THE REST OF THE VCFS PHENOTYPE?

In the context of pronounced cognitive deficits, it is important to mention that delays in motor coordination are likely to affect certain cognitive tests, especially those measuring processing speed and manipulation of materials. Motor delays have been consistently observed in the syndrome, among preschool (Gerdes, Solot, Wang, McDonald-McGinn, & Zackai, 2001; Gerdes et al., 1999) and school-age children (Swillen et al., 1999). Fine motor skills, including motor dexterity through finger tapping, kinesthetic awareness through imitating hand positions, and graphomotor control, were recently shown to be impaired in affected school-age individuals (Sobin et al., 2005). Although all three forms of motor control were delayed compared to other cognitive skills, motor control was not associated with a measure of visuo-spatial memory. This suggests that, despite manipulation demands during certain visuo-spatial tasks, motor delays do not entirely explain visuo-spatial difficulties in VCFS.

Affected individuals also consistently report difficulties estimating time, a difficulty that may be related to both slowed processing and a lack of motor fluidity. A recent study demonstrated that individuals with the syndrome have difficulties reproducing temporal intervals and judging the difference in the presentation lengths of auditory and visual stimuli. Affected individuals required a greater disparity between the lengths of two presentations in order to accurately detect a difference. Further, affected individuals varied more than controls in their reproductions of an auditory rhythm and left less time between sounds (Debbane, Glaser, Gex-Fabry, & Eliez, 2005).

Reductions of the cerebellum and the parietal lobe are implicated in the motor problems in VCFS, given that both regions are reduced (Eliez et al., 2002; van Amelsvoort et al., 2001). However, it now seems that motor impairments may be specifically related to dysfunction in a brain circuit called the cortico-cerebellar-thalamic-cortical circuit (Figures 3–2 and 3–3), which is linked to a disruption in the fluidity of thoughts and actions known as cognitive dysmetria (Andreasen, 1999). Automatic motor adjustments, the fluidity and flow of cognitive processing required for accurate temporal perception, as well as the discontinuity between thoughts observed in schizophrenia, all have been attributed to this circuit (Andreasen, 1999). Taken together, studies of VCFS present a similar pattern of disruption through evidence for deficits in temporal perception (Debbane et al., 2005), motor difficulties (Gerdes et al., 2001; Gerdes et al., 1999; Sobin et al., 2005), an elevated risk for psychosis (Murphy, 2005), and attention problems (see above section). Moreover, neuroanatomical studies have hypothesized decreased cortico-thalamic connectivity in the VCFS brain (Barnea-Goraly et al., 2003; Schaer et al., 2005; T. J. Simon, Ding, et al., 2005) through decreased white matter and inter-regional connectivity (Barnea-Goraly et al., 2003; Kates et al., 2001; T. J. Simon,

Ding, et al., 2005), decreased cerebellar volumes, and decreased thalamic volumes (Bish et al., 2004). Clearly, such a disruption in the flow of processing and motor movements impacts a child's learning curve and level of functioning. For this reason, it is important to take sensorimotor difficulties into consideration when planning for a child's educational program.

This chapter has attempted to shed light on some of the major cognitive weaknesses associated with VCFS, as well as the brain changes that may underlie these weaknesses. Although alterations to complex circuits in the VCFS brain contribute to several, or all, of the aforementioned abilities, they have been discussed separately so as to be the most applicable to educational interventions. One unifying goal of the many studies mentioned in this chapter is to inform educational programs and clinical treatments for affected persons. Indeed, years of research have demonstrated the broad impact that a child's educational environment and teachers have on his knowledge, attention, relationships, and empathy. To optimize the school environment of a child with VCFS, it seems essential to take into account the major learning difficulties associated with the syndrome, as well as his individual needs.

# REFERENCES

Adolphs, R. (2003). Cognitive neuroscience of human social behaviour. *Nature Reviews Neuroscience, 4,* 165–178.

Adolphs, R., Tranel, D., & Buchanan, T. W. (2005). Amygdala damage impairs emotional memory for gist but not details of complex stimuli. *Nature Neuroscience, 8,* 512–518.

Andreasen, N. C. (1999). A unitary model of schizophrenia: Bleuler's "fragmented phrene" as schizencephaly. *Archives of General Psychiatry, 56,* 781–787.

Baker, K. D., & Skuse, D. H. (2005). Adolescents and young adults with 22q11 deletion syndrome: Psychopathology in an at-risk group. *British Journal of Psychiatry, 186,* 115–120.

Barnea-Goraly, N., Eliez, S., Menon, V., Bammer, R., & Reiss, A. L. (2005). Arithmetic ability and parietal alterations: A diffusion tensor imaging study in velocardiofacial syndrome. *Brain Research. Cognitive Brain Research, 25,* 735–740.

Barnea-Goraly, N., Menon, V., Krasnow, B., Ko, A., Reiss, A., & Eliez, S. (2003). Investigation of white matter structure in velocardiofacial syndrome: A diffusion tensor imaging study. *American Journal of Psychiatry, 160,* 1863–1869.

Bearden, C. E., Woodin, M. F., Wang P. P., Moss, E., McDonald-McGinn, D., Zackai, E., et al. (2001). The neurocognitive phenotype of the 22q11.2 deletion syndrome: Selective deficit in visual-spatial memory. *Journal of Clinical Experimental Neuropsychology, 23,* 447–464.

Bellugi, U., Lichtenberger, L., Jones, W., Lai, Z., & St. George, M. I. (2000). The neurocognitive profile of Williams syndrome: A complex pattern of strengths and weaknesses. *Journal of Cognitive Neuroscience, 12*(Suppl. 1), 7–29.

Bish, J. P., Ferrante, S. M., McDonald-McGinn, D., Zackai, E., & Simon, T. J. (2005). Maladaptive conflict monitoring as evidence for executive dysfunction in children with chromosome 22q11.2 deletion syndrome. *Developmental Science, 8,* 36–43.

Bish, J. P., Nguyen, V., Ding, L., Ferrante, S., & Simon, T. J. (2004). Thalamic reductions in children with chromosome 22q11.2 deletion syndrome. *Neuroreport, 15,* 1413–1415.

Chow, E. W., Zipursky, R. B., Mikulis, D. J., & Bassett, A.S. (2002). Structural brain abnormalities in patients with schizophrenia and 22q11 deletion syndrome. *Biological Psychiatry, 51,* 208–215.

De Smedt, B., Ghesquiere, P., & Swillen, A. (2005). Mathematical disabilities in genetic syndromes: The case of velo-cardio-facial syndrome. In F. Columbus (Ed.), *Learning disabilities: New research.* New York: Nova Publishers.

De Smedt, B., Swillen, A., Ghesquiere, P., Devriendt, K., & Fryns, J. P. (2003). Pre-academic and early academic achievement in children with velocardiofacial syndrome (del22q11.2) of borderline or normal intelligence. *Genetetic Counseling, 14,* 15–29.

Debbane, M., Glaser, B., Gex-Fabry ,M., & Eliez, S. (2005). Temporal perception in velo-cardio-facial syndrome. *Neuropsychologia, 43,* 1754–1762.

Eliez, S., Barnea-Goraly, N., Schmitt, J. E., Liu, Y., & Reiss, A. L. (2002). Increased basal ganglia volumes in velo-cardio-facial syndrome (deletion 22q11.2). *Biological Psychiatry, 52,* 68–70.

Eliez, S., Blasey, C. M., Menon, V., White, C. D., Schmitt, J. E., & Reiss, A, L. (2001). Functional brain imaging study of mathematical reasoning abilities in velocardiofacial syndrome (del22q11.2). *Genetic Medicine, 3,* 49–55.

Eliez, S., Blasey, C. M., Schmitt, E. J., White, C. D., Hu, D., & Reiss, A. L. (2001). Velocardiofacial syndrome: Are structural changes in the temporal and mesial temporal regions related to schizophrenia? *American Journal of Psychiatry, 158,* 447–453.

Eliez, S., Schmitt, J. E., White, C. D., Wellis, V. G., & Reiss, A. L. (2001). A quantitative MRI study of posterior fossa development in velocardiofacial syndrome. *Biological Psychiatry, 49,* 540–546.

Feinstein, C., Eliez, S., Blasey, C., & Reiss, A. L. (2002). Psychiatric disorders and behavioral problems in children with velocardiofacial syndrome: Usefulness as phenotypic indicators of schizophrenia risk. *Biological Psychiatry, 51,* 312–318.

Gerdes, M., Solot, C., Wang, P. P., McDonald-McGinn, D. M., & Zackai, E. H. (2001). Taking advantage of early diagnosis: Preschool children with the 22q11.2 deletion. *Genetic Medicine, 3,* 40–44.

Gerdes, M., Solot, C., Wang, P. P., Moss, E., LaRossa, D., Randall, P., et al. (1999). Cognitive and behavior profile of preschool children with chromosome 22q11.2 deletion. *American Journal of Medical Genetics, 85,* 127–133.

Giedd, J. N., Blumenthal, J., Jeffries, N. O., Castellanos, F. X., Liu, H., Zijdenbos, A., et al. (1999). Brain development during childhood and adolescence: A longitudinal MRI study. *Nature Neuroscience, 2,* 861–863.

Glaser, B., Mumme, D. L., Blasey, C., Morris, M. A., Dahoun, S. P., Antonarakis, S. E., et al. (2002). Language skills in children with velocardiofacial syndrome (deletion 22q11.2). *Journal of Pediatrics, 140,* 753–758.

Golding-Kushner, K. J., Weller, G., & Shprintzen, R. J. (1985). Velo-cardio-facial syndrome: Language and psychological profiles. *Journal of Craniofacial Genetics and Developmental Biology, 5,* 259–266.

Gothelf, D., Eliez, S., Thompson, T., Hinard, C., Penniman, L., Feinstein, C., et al. (2005). COMT genotype predicts longitudinal cognitive decline and psychosis in 22q11.2 deletion syndrome. *Nature Neuroscience, 8,* 1500–1502.

Gothelf, D., Gruber, R., Presburger, G., Dotan, I., Brand-Gothelf, A., Burg, M., et al. (2003). Methylphenidate treatment for attention-deficit/hyperactivity disorder in children and adolescents with velocardiofacial syndrome: An open-label study. *Journal of Clinical Psychiatry, 64,* 1163–1169.

Gothelf, D., Presburger, G., Levy, D., Nahmani, A., Burg, M., Berant, M., et al. (2004). Genetic, developmental, and physical factors associated with attention deficit hyperactivity disorder in patients with velocardiofacial syndrome. *American Journal of Medical Genetics. Part B, Neuropsychiatric Genetics, 126,* 116–121.

Haxby, J. V., Gobbini, M. I., Furey, M. L., Ishai, A., Schouten, J. L., & Pietrini, P. (2001). Distributed and overlapping representations of faces and objects in ventral temporal cortex. *Science, 293,* 2425–2430.

Haxby, J. V., Hoffman, E. A., & Gobbini, M.I. (2000). The distributed human neural system for face perception. *Trends in Cognitive Science, 4,* 223–233.

Henry, J. C., van Amelsvoort, T., Morris, R. G., Owen, M. J., Murphy, D. G. M., & Murphy, K. C. (2002). An investigation of the neuropsychological profile in adults with velo-cardio-facial syndrome (VCFS). *Neuropsychologia, 40,* 471–478.

Hubbard, E. M., Piazza, M., Pinel, P., & Dehaene, S. (2005). Interactions between number and space in parietal cortex. *Nature Reviews Neuroscience, 6,* 435–448.

Johnson, M. H. (2005). Subcortical face processing. *Nature Reviews Neuroscience, 6,* 766–774.

Johnson, M. H, Dziurawiec, S., Ellis, H., & Morton, J. (1991). Newborns' preferential tracking of face-like stimuli and its subsequent decline. *Cognition, 40,* 1–19.

Kanwisher, N., McDermott, J., & Chun, M. M. (1997). The fusiform face area: A module in human extrastriate cortex specialized for face perception. *Journal of Neuroscience, 17,* 4302–4311.

Kates, W. R., Antshel, K., Willhite, R., Bessette, B. A., AbdulSabur, N., & Higgins, A. M. (2005). Gender-moderated dorsolateral prefrontal reductions in 22q11.2 deletion syndrome: Implications for risk for schizophrenia. *Child Neuropsychology, 11,* 73–85.

Kates, W. R., Burnette, C. P., Jabs, E. W., Rutberg, J., Murphy, A. M., Grados, M., et al. (2001). Regional cortical white matter reductions in velocardiofacial syndrome: A volumetric MRI analysis. *Biological Psychiatry, 49,* 677–684.

Kok, L. L., & Solman, R. T. (1995). Velocardiofacial syndrome: Learning difficulties and intervention. *Journal of Medical Genetics, 32,* 612–618.

Majerus, S., Glaser, B., Van der Linden, M., & Eliez, S. (2006). A multiple case study of verbal short-term memory in velo-cardio-facial syndrome. *Journal of Intellectual Disability Research, 50*(Pt. 6), 457–469.

Milner, A. D., & Goodale, M. A. (1995). *The visual brain in action.* Oxford: Oxford University Press.

Mishkin, M., & Ungerleider, L. G. (1982). Contribution of striate inputs to the visuospatial functions of parieto-preoccipital cortex in monkeys. *Behavioral Brain Research, 6,* 57–77.

Monchi, O., Petrides, M., Strafella, A. P., Worsley, K. J., & Doyon, J. (2006). Functional role of the basal ganglia in the planning and execution of actions. *Annals of Neurology, 59,* 257–264.

Mondloch, C. J., Geldart, S., Maurer, D., & Le Grand, R. (2003). Developmental changes in face processing skills. *Journal of Experimental Child Psychology, 86,* 67–84.

Moss, E. M., Batshaw, M. L., Solot, C. B., Gerdes, M., McDonald-McGinn, D. M., Driscoll, D. A., et al. (1999). Psychoeducational profile of the 22q11.2 microdeletion: A complex pattern. *Journal of Pediatrics, 134,* 193–198.

Murphy, K. C. (2005). Annotation: Velo-cardio-facial syndrome. *Journal of Child Psychology and Psychiatry*, *46*, 563–571.

Niklasson, L., Rasmussen, P., Oskarsdottir, S., & Gillberg, C. (2001). Neuropsychiatric disorders in the 22q11 deletion syndrome. *Genetic Medicine*, *3*, 79–84.

Paterson, S. J., Girelli, L., Butterworth, B., & Karmiloff-Smith, A. (2006). Are numerical impairments syndrome specific? Evidence from Williams syndrome and Down's syndrome. *Journal of Child Psychology and Psychiatry*, *47*, 190–204.

Posner, M. I., & Petersen, S. E. (1990). The attention system of the human brain. *Annual Review of Neuroscience*, *13*, 25–42.

Reiss, A. L., Abrams, M. T., Singer, H. S., Ross, J. L., & Denckla, M. B. (1996). Brain development, gender and IQ in children. A volumetric imaging study. *Brain*, *119* (Pt. 5), 1763–1774.

Schaer, M., Schmitt, J. E., Glaser, B., Lazeyras, F., Delavelle, J., & Eliez, S. (2005). Abnormal patterns of cortical gyrification in velo-cardio-facial syndrome (deletion 22q11.2): An MRI study. *Psychiatry Research*, *146*, 1–11.

Scherer, N. J., D'Antonio, L. L., & Kalbfleisch, J. H. (1999). Early speech and language development in children with velocardiofacial syndrome. *American Journal of Medical Genetics*, *88*, 714–723.

Schmahmann, J. D. (2004). Disorders of the cerebellum: Ataxia, dysmetria of thought, and the cerebellar cognitive affective syndrome. *Journal of Neuropsychiatry and Clinical Neuroscience*, *16*, 367–378.

Seidman, L. J., Valera, E. M., & Makris, N. (2005). Structural brain imaging of attention-deficit/hyperactivity disorder. *Biological Psychiatry*, *57*, 1263–1272.

Shashi, V., Muddasani, S., Santos, C. C., Berry, M. N., Kwapil, T. R., Lewandowski, E., et al. (2004). Abnormalities of the corpus callosum in nonpsychotic children with chromosome 22q11 deletion syndrome. *Neuroimage*, *21*, 1399–1406.

Shprintzen R. J. (2005). Velo-cardio-facial syndrome. *Progress in Pediatric Cardiology*, *20*, 187–193.

Simon, O., Kherif, F., Flandin, G., Poline, J. B., Riviere, D., Mangin, J. F., et al. (2004). Automatized clustering and functional geometry of human parietofrontal networks for language, space, and number. *Neuroimage*, *23*, 1192–1202.

Simon, T. J., Bearden, C. E., McGinn, D. M., & Zackai, E. (2005). Visuospatial and numerical cognitive deficits in children with chromosome 22q11.2 deletion syndrome. *Cortex*, *41*, 145–155.

Simon, T. J., Bish, J. P., Bearden, C. E., Ding, L., Ferrante, S., Nguyen, V., et al. (2005). A multilevel analysis of cognitive dysfunction and psychopathology associated with chromosome 22q11.2 deletion syndrome in children. *Developmental Psychopathology*, *17*, 753–784.

Simon, T. J., Ding, L., Bish, J. P., McDonald-McGinn, D. M., Zackai, E. H., & Gee, J. (2005). Volumetric, connective, and morphologic changes in the brains of children with chromosome 22q11.2 deletion syndrome: An integrative study. *Neuroimage*, *25*, 169–180.

Sobin, C., Kiley-Brabeck, K., Daniels, S., Blundell, M., Anyane-Yeboa, K., & Karayiorgou, M. (2004). Networks of attention in children with the 22q11 deletion syndrome. *Developmental Neuropsychology*, *26*, 611–626.

Sobin, C., Kiley-Brabeck, K., Daniels, S., Khuri, J., Taylor, L., Blundell, M., et al. (2005). Neuropsychological characteristics of children with the 22q11 deletion syndrome: A descriptive analysis. *Child Neuropsychology*, *11*, 39–53.

Solot, C. B., Gerdes, M., Kirschner, R. E., McDonald-McGinn, D. M., Moss, E., Woodin, M., et al. (2001). Communication issues in 22q11.2 deletion syndrome: Children at risk. *Genetic Medicine*, *3*, 67–71.

Solot, C. B., Knightly, C., Handler, S. D., Gerdes, M., McDonald-McGinn, D. M., Moss, E., et al. (2000). Communication disorders in the 22q11.2 microdeletion syndrome. *Journal of Communication Disorders*, *33*, 187–203; quiz 203–204.

Swillen, A., Devriendt, K., Legius, E., Eyskens, B., Dumoulin, M., Gewillig, M., et al. (1997). Intelligence and psychosocial adjustment in velocardiofacial syndrome: A study of 37 children and adolescents with VCFS. *Journal of Medical Genetics*, *34*, 453–458.

Swillen, A., Vandeputte, L., Cracco, J., Maes, B., Ghesquiere, P., Devriendt, K., et al. (1999). Neuropsychological, learning and psychosocial profile of primary school aged children with the velo-cardio-facial syndrome (22q11 deletion): Evidence for a nonverbal learning disability? *Child Neuropsychology*, *5*, 230–241.

van Amelsvoort, T., Daly, E., Henry, J., Robertson, D., Ng, V., Owen, M., et al. (2004). Brain anatomy in adults with velocardiofacial syndrome with and without schizophrenia: Preliminary results of a structural magnetic resonance imaging study. *Archives of General Psychiatry*, *61*, 1085–1096.

van Amelsvoort, T., Daly, E., Robertson, D., Suckling, J., Ng, V., Critchley, H., et al. (2001). Structural brain abnormalities associated with deletion at chromosome 22q11: Quantitative neuroimaging study of adults with velo-cardio-facial syndrome. *British Journal of Psychiatry*, *178*, 412–419.

van Amelsvoort, T., Henry, J., Morris, R., Owen, M., Linszen, D., Murphy, K., et al. (2004). Cognitive deficits associated with schizophrenia in velo-cardio-facial syndrome. *Schizophrenia Research*, *70*, 223–232.

Vuilleumier, P., Armony, J. L., Driver, J., & Dolan, R. J. (2003). Distinct spatial frequency sensitivies for processing faces and emotional expressions. *Nature Neuroscience*, *6*, 624–631.

Wang, P. P., Woodin, M. F., Kreps-Falk, R., & Moss, E. M. (2000). Research on behavioral phenotypes: Velocardiofacial syndrome (deletion 22q11.2). *Developmental Medicine & Child Neurology*, *42*, 422–427.

Wilke, M., Sohn, J. H., Byars, A. W., & Holland, S. K. (2003). Bright spots: Correlations of gray matter volume with IQ in a normal pediatric population. *Neuroimage*, *20*, 202–215.

Woodin, M., Wang, P. P., Aleman, D., McDonald-McGinn, D., Zackai, E., & Moss, E. (2001). Neuropsychological profile of children and adolescents with the 22q11.2 microdeletion. *Genetic Medicine*, *3*, 34–39.

Zinkstok, J., & van Amelsvoort, T. (2005). Neuropsychological profile and neuroimaging in patients with 22q11.2 deletion syndrome: A review. *Child Neuropsychology*, *11*, 21–37.

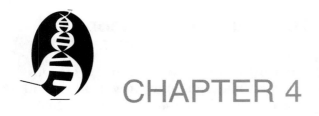

CHAPTER 4

# Psychiatric Disorders and Treatment in Velo-Cardio-Facial Syndrome

### DORON GOTHELF, MD
### MERAV BURG, MA

$V$elo-cardio-facial syndrome (VCFS) seems to be a model of abnormal neuropsychiatric development that manifests in milder psychiatric symptoms during early childhood and in about one-third of the subjects it escalates to psychosis by young adulthood (Bassett et al., 1998; Feinstein, Eliez, Blasey, & Reiss, 2002; Murphy, Jones, & Owen, 1999; Shprintzen, 2000). Teachers are in a pivotal position to identify early signs of distress in children with VCFS and thus need to know the signs suggesting that the child should be referred for psychiatric evaluation. In this chapter we will describe the common emotional challenges and psychiatric disorders that characterize individuals with VCFS. These will be divided into the common disorders and deficits that are manifested already during childhood and the schizophrenia-like psychotic disorder that evolves during adolescence and young adulthood. At the last part of the chapter we will describe the psychological and medication treatment modalities for this population.

## MANIFESTATIONS BEGINNING IN CHILDHOOD

Already in preschool years children with VCFS are often described as anxious, shy, withdrawn, stubborn, emotionally labile, and afflicted with social and communication impairments (Swillen, Devriendt, Ghesquiere, & Fryns, 2001). In general, it seems that most of the emotional and psychiatric issues that children with VCFS are facing are not unique or specific to the syndrome. A similar psychiatric profile of social deficits, low self-esteem, and increased rate of a variety of psychiatric disorders is common to children with heterogeneous causes of developmental disabilities and to children coping with other chronic medical conditions (Dykens, 2000; Geist, Grdisa, & Otley, 2003).

### Deficits in Social Skills

Similarly to other children with developmental disabilities, children with VCFS commonly suffer from social incompetence and immature social skills. The social incompetence is caused by their difficulties in understanding social situations and by a limited repertoire of social skills (Swillen et al., 1999). Consequently children with VCFS encounter extreme difficulties in establishing and maintaining peer relationships. Like most children they very much want to be accepted by their peers; however, they tend to withdraw from social activities and to be isolated and lonely. Often parents are concerned with the fact that, although the children express a wish for social belonging, at the same time they are very limited in their ability to take part in social activities. The deficient or ineffective social skills of children and adolescents with VCFS are apparent in several aspects. They tend to be shy and avoidant during social interactions. Some of them have difficulties to predict consequences of certain social behaviors and are more likely to choose socially unacceptable behaviors, such as being the class clown or behaving on purpose in a very childish-regressive way.

Recently it has been reported that children with VCFS have an increased rate of autism spectrum disorders (Fine et al., 2005). It is important to note that in general children with developmental disabilities have social skill deficits. Although there are exceptions, in general the more retarded a child is, the more profound are his social deficits (Bielecki & Swender, 2004; Wing & Gould, 1979). Since the studies that reported autism spectrum disorders in VCFS did not have a matched IQ control group it is still not certain whether autism is specifically associated with VCFS.

Lack of assertiveness is a source of constant frustration in the social interaction of children with VCFS. The lack of assertiveness is manifested in their impaired ability to resist peer pressure, to give and accept criticism, and to negotiate their needs appropriately. The lack of assertiveness also commonly leads to oppositional behaviors, which are often more severe at home towards parents than at school. Often the teacher and peers experience the child as a quiet and obedient child while at home the child expresses his frustration by behaving appositionally towards his parents and siblings (Swillen et al., 1999).

## Low Self-Esteem

Low self-esteem and negative self-perception are very common in individuals with VCFS (Burg & Gothelf, 2003). There are several risk factors that contribute to their low self-esteem including the learning disabilities, medical handicaps, hypernasal speech, and psychiatric disorders. Often children with VCFS avoid participating in academic activities because they are concerned with their poor reading and poor schoolwork performance and are afraid that their classmates will make fun of them. Children with VCFS tend to keep away from sports games; oftentimes they are the last to be chosen for team games and as a consequence they prefer to watch passively instead of participating. Most children with VCFS are not satisfied with their appearance. They are preoccupied with the special facial features related to the syndrome and dislike their hypernasal speech. Some of the children tend to cope with this negative physical self-perception by neglecting their physical appearance. The negative self-perception can also affect their relations with parents. Often children with VCFS feel that parents are disappointed with them and they perceive themselves as a source of constant problems and hardship to their families. They also tend to compare their social and academic achievements with those of their siblings, which often leads them to develop serious doubts about their own self-worth.

## Psychiatric Disorders

As stated previously, all children with developmental disabilities, including VCFS, have a high rate of psychiatric disorders (Dykens, 2000; Feinstein et al., 2002; Geist et al., 2003). Feinstein et al. (2002) compared the rate of psychiatric disorders in children and adolescents with VCFS with that of matched IQ controls and found similar very high rates of psychiatric disorders in both groups. Swillen et al. (2001) compared parents' and teachers' reports of the behavior of school-aged children with VCFS with reports of matched age and IQ controls with speech and language impairments but without VCFS. The results indicated that overall both groups exhibited similar degrees of abnormal behaviors. It is not surprising that children with developmental disabilities have similarly high rates of behavioral problems and psychiatric disorders because they share common risk factors for psychopathology, such as social isolation and rejection, impairments in social and daily living skills, low self-esteem, and overprotectiveness by parents. These factors could predispose them to psychiatric morbidity.

The most common psychiatric disorder in children with VCFS is attention-deficit hyperactivity disorder (ADHD) present in 40–50% of children with VCFS (Arnold, Siegel-Bartelt, Cytrynbaum, Teshima, & Schachar, 2001; Gothelf et al., 2003; Papolos et al., 1996). The inattentive symptoms (such as difficulty sustaining attention or with organization skills) are usually more frequent in individuals with VCFS than the hyperactive symptoms (such as motor restless-ness) (Gothelf et al., 2003). In contrast to the hyperactive symptoms, inatten-tive symptoms are easily missed because they may not be disruptive to the classroom or home environment. Clinical evaluation of ADHD symptoms in children with cognitive deficits is challenging. The teachers and clinicians should consider the mental age of the child and not the chronological age. In the case of VCFS, the mental age is frequently lagging two to four years behind their chronological age (Shprintzen, 2000). Hence, for example expectations regarding the time span they can concentrate should be gauged accordingly. Inattention should also be distinguished from inability of the child to follow a school program that is too difficult for his or her academic level, especially for those children with VCFS who are studying in the mainstream.

Some abnormal behaviors seen in children with VCFS frequently do not fit the diagnostic entities defined by the psychiatric classification DSM-IV-TR nomenclature. A prototypic example is the repetitive-stereotypic behaviors that are very common in children with VCFS and which could be defined as obsessive-compulsive disorder (OCD). OCD has been reported to occur in up to almost one-third of individuals with VCFS (Gothelf et al., 2004). The OCD symptoms included rituals related to excessive washing and cleaning, hoard-ing, and somatic worries (Gothelf et al., 2004). However, the presentation of OCD in children with VCFS is different in several aspects from the OCD seen in adults or in typically developing children. First, the presence of obsessions is far less common in VCFS. In addition, children with VCFS tend not to try to resist the compulsions and often do not recognize their abnormal nature, and thus usually they have a low motivation to change their compulsive habits. One of the most common compulsive habits of children with VCFS is repeti-tive questions (Gothelf et al., 2004). Often the questions are related to excit-ing events that the child is looking forward to such as going with the parents to buy a toy in a shop. The child in this case will repetitively and relentlessly ask his parents, "When are we going to the store?" It seems that a common theme in many of the repetitive questions is the time of the events that the child is looking forward to or is anxious about. Children with VCFS may be especially preoccupied with time because their time perception is impaired (Debbane, Glaser, Gex-Fabry, & Eliez, 2005). Repetitive questions and other repetitive behaviors are common in children with other genetic syndromes (e.g., Williams syndrome and Prader-Willi syndrome) and in children with other developmental disabilities such as autism spectrum disorders (Dykens, Leckman, & Cassidy, 1996; Mervis and Klein-Tasman, 2000). Because these repetitive behaviors are not commonly seen in typically developing children with OCD, some clinicians define them as perseverative or stereotypic behav-iors rather than OCD.

## Case Vignette #1

A 12-year-old boy had tetralogy of Fallot and hypernasal speech due to velo-pharyngeal insufficiency. His IQ was 65, and he attended special education classes. Psychiatric diagnoses included OCD, ADHD, and dog, cat, and noise phobias. He was afraid of being infected by bacteria and refrained from using plates and cutlery that he suspected had been touched by another person. At the time of the study, he was preoccupied with his bar mitzvah ceremony and repeatedly asked his parents questions about it: where it was going to be held; the number of steps in the hall; the availability of a guest elevator so that handicapped children could participate. He was also very preoccupied with time and hoarded clocks. Every hour on the hour, he counted to 10 and stretched. He tended to rock each leg an even number of times, and constantly rearranged his cupboard until it felt "just right."

Besides OCD, children with VCFS tend to have a high rate of other anxiety disorders including generalized anxiety, separation anxiety, and phobias (Feinstein et al., 2002; Gothelf et al., 2004). They worry excessively about all manner of upcoming events and occurrences. The anxiety can be about separation from parents, their own health, something catastrophic happening, being judged, or social situations. During preschool and elementary school years often separation from a parent is difficult for children with VCFS. They tend to cling to their parent and have trouble falling asleep by themselves at night. When separated, they may fear that their parent will be involved in an accident or be taken ill, or that they will "lose" him in some other way. Because of their need to stay close to their parent or home they may refrain from going on school trips or to camps, staying at friends' houses, or being in a room by themselves. As they grow older this problem becomes more serious and demanding. The parents may feel that they are forced to change their daily routine in order to be near their anxious child and the child or adolescent himself feels incapable of doing ordinary things like his siblings or peers.

Another aspect of the anxious predisposition of children with VCFS is their shyness that is frequently manifested as social phobia. Usually the problem begins very early when the child learns to speak. In the case of VCFS, many children suffer from hypernasal speech that is difficult to comprehend (Shprint-zen et al., 1978). They receive negative feedback from other children and teachers who fail to comprehend their communication. Children also often mock the speech of a child with VCFS. As a result, children with VCFS tend to refrain from speaking to people outside the close family. After the speech is corrected by surgery they usually "open to the world" and begin to be more talkative and social but, in many cases, the inhibited nature still persists. Children with VCFS are afraid of being embarrassed in social situations, during a performance, or if they have to speak in class or in public. They feel anxious while being introduced to other people, or while talking with others, or while interacting with people in authority. Being watched or observed while eating, drinking, or writing in public could be embarrassing as well. In social interactions, children with VCFS tend to be quiet, backward, withdrawn, and inhibited. They might seem unfriendly, aloof, and disinterested, but at the same time, they really want to take part and be socially accepted. The social phobia causes distress and misery to the child and his family. Many children with VCFS try to avoid social interactions with children of their age and prefer to spend time at home with their parents rather then interacting with peers.

### Case Vignette #2

Tamara, 12 years old, is the second child to a family of five that lives in a small village in the center of Israel. Tamara was diagnosed with VCFS when she was 7 years old. From a medical standpoint, she was born with a tetralogy of Fallot (TOF) heart defect, underwent surgery at age 2, and is currently under cardiological surveillance. Tamara was born with a cleft palate and underwent surgery when she was 7, yet the palate is still susceptible to nasalization. She suffers from a slight curvature of the spine and is due to undergo surgery in the future. Her facial features are reflective of her syndrome, and she appears small for her age. Tamara's intellectual capability falls on the lower end of the normal range. She reads and writes well. However, she has difficulty in reading comprehension and her mathematical understanding is low. She requires parental help in doing homework and getting ready for school. In the past, Tamara learned in a regular school in the village in which she lives. Due to difficulties in academic as well as social integration, Tamara moved to another regular education school in a city close by, two years ago. The class size in Tamara's new school is small. Tamara's parents sought psychological counseling when Tamara was 10 years old. They reported that Tamara has many fears that cause her and her family much distress. Tamara refuses to take the school bus in the mornings from fear that the other children will bother her and laugh at her. She often calls her parents from school and asks that they take her home. She does not leave the house in the afternoons yet has difficulty occupying herself. She feels lonely and is jealous of her siblings who are socially active. At times, she picks fights with them. Tamara avoids speaking with people who are not close family members. She is very dependent upon her parents, in particular, in all areas of daily functioning. Upon examination, Tamara was diagnosed as having social phobia. She suspects that others will criticize her and mock her. She is disturbed about her outer appearance and has a low self-image. She often compares herself with her siblings and classmates, and feels less talented and less beautiful than they. Because of her fear of meeting pupils every outing, be it to the shopping mall, hairdresser, or yard, involves much suffering and anxiety.

Besides anxiety disorders children and adolescents with VCFS have an increased rate of affective disorders, especially depression (Feinstein et al., 2002). Mood swings are very common in VCFS and one study reported that as high as two-thirds of children with VCFS have a bipolar affective disorder (Papolos et al.,

1996). Other studies, however, did not observe such a high rate of bipolar affective disorder in VCFS. Our experience is that indeed mood swings are common in VCFS but they are usually a part of ADHD or oppositional behavior. Children with VCFS do not usually manifest other symptoms required for the diagnosis of a manic episode such as megalomanic thoughts, increased energy, decreased need for sleep, and racing thoughts.

## MANIFESTATIONS DURING ADOLESCENCE

In a recent longitudinal study, children with VCFS and matched IQ control children were first evaluated during preadolescence and then reevaluated at late adolescence–early adulthood (Gothelf et al., 2005). The study found that at baseline, during preadolescence, the two groups had a similar high rate of psychiatric disorders including ADHD and anxiety and depressive disorders (Feinstein et al., 2002). At follow-up, during late adolescence–early adulthood, the control subjects significantly improved in terms of rate of anxiety and depressive disorders and social functioning. In VCFS, in contrast, the rate of anxiety and depressive disorders remained high and social deficits became more prominent (Gothelf et al., in press). In addition, 32% of the adolescents and young adults developed a psychotic disorder (Gothelf et al., 2005).

Other studies with VCFS population have also reported that 25% of subjects develop schizophrenia-like psychotic disorder by early adulthood (Murphy et al., 1999). The age of onset of the psychotic disorder varies from as low as the age of 10 years to as high as 25 years. The clinical characteristics of the VCFS psychotic disorder are similar to those of schizophrenia patients from the general population (Bassett et al., 2003). The strong association between VCFS and schizophrenia-like psychosis does indeed seem to be specific because the rate of schizophrenia in VCFS is about 25 times more common than in the general population and about 10 times more common than in individuals with other developmental disabilities (Turner, 1989). The extremely high rate of schizophrenia in VCFS makes the syndrome the most common known genetic risk factor to schizophrenia. The risk is higher even than being an offspring of a patient with schizophrenia (Murphy, 2002). It seems plausible that the psychosis in VCFS is the result of one or more genes that are missing in these subjects. One of the genes in the VCFS deletion region is the COMT gene. The COMT gene codes for the COMT enzyme that is responsible for degradation of dopamine. High brain dopamine levels induce psychotic symptoms and all antipsychotic medications reduce brain dopamine activity. Thus the deficiency in COMT seems a plausible mechanism for the risk of psychosis in VCFS. One study found that those VCFS subjects with an extreme shortage of COMT (subjects with VCFS carrying the low activity allele) are at especially increased risk for decline in verbal cognitive abilities and the development of psychotic symptoms (Gothelf et al., 2005).

Another longitudinal investigation of the same cohort of subjects found that having subthreshold psychotic symptoms during childhood was a risk factor for developing a full-blown psychotic disorder (Gothelf et al., in press). Thus, when a child with VCFS reports about hallucinations or thoughts that seems unrealistic (delusions) he or she should be referred for evaluation. In addition, the study found that the presence of anxiety disorders, and especially OCD, also was a risk factor for the later development of a psychotic disorder (Gothelf et al., in press).

Infants and toddlers with VCFS that suffer from severe physical diseases are usually identified by clinicians and referred for genetic testing at infancy and preschool years. Those that are only mildly physically affected are easily missed. Clinicians should be alert to adolescents that manifest marked cognitive limitations and psychiatric symptoms, especially psychotic symptoms, and refer them for a genetic testing for VCFS.

### Case Vignette #3

Nathalie, a 17 year-old female, was hospitalized at a psychiatric inpatient unit after threatening to commit suicide and becoming physically violent toward her parents. On psychiatric evaluation she reported delusions of reference thinking that her classmates and even strangers in the street were saying "nasty things" about her. She also reported that figures from the TV were telling her how ugly she was. Nathalie also reported that she heard voices telling her to commit suicide, and her parents noted that she was talking to herself loudly as if arguing with someone. The psychiatrist diagnosed Nathalie with schizoaffective disorder, depressive type. Nathalie is otherwise a relatively physically healthy adolescent. She was born with mild ventricular septal defect that closed spontaneously. Her attainment of developmental milestones was slightly delayed but within the normal range and she had mild hypotonia as a young child. Her speech was mildly hypernasal. In elementary school she had difficulties with mathematics and reading comprehension. Cognitive testing showed that Nathalie's IQ was 78. In elementary school Nathalie was also diagnosed with ADHD inattentive type and suffered from anxiety disorders. She used to cling to her parents and refused to go on a trip or to visit friends without being accompanied by her parents. At the age of 12 years she also started having compulsions in which she repetitively touched her eye to make sure she would not develop strabismus, and she compulsively hoarded paper, magazines, and advertisements and would not let anyone touch the collection. The combination of her psychiatric symptoms with a history of ventricular septal defect, hypernasal speech, and mild dysmorphic facial features raised her psychiatrist's suspicion that Nathalie might have VCFS. Nathalie was referred for a FISH test, and the result was positive for the 22q11.2 deletion. Nathalie is an example of a physically healthy child with mild developmental delay but with severe psychiatric symptomatology. Nathalie's psychiatric disorders were first noticed in elementary school and gradually escalated. Initially, ADHD developed, followed by separation anxiety disorder and OCD, culminating at the age of 17 years with a psychotic disorder. Since Nathalie's physical symptoms were very mild and included only a VSD and hypernasal speech, her diagnosis could have been easily missed. Of the myriad psychiatric symptoms that Nathalie had, the schizophrenia-like symptoms were the ones that were relatively specific to VCFS. Thus it was the combination of psychotic symptoms, the few physical symptoms characteristic of the syndrome, and the borderline intelligence that raised the clinical suspicion that Nathalie may be affected with VCFS.

## PSYCHOSOCIAL AND PSYCHIATRIC TREATMENTS IN VCFS

The ultimate goal is to develop specific treatments to the cognitive deficits and neuropsychiatric disorders of individuals with VCFS. However, we still do not know enough about the biological and environmental factors that interact to induce these deficits and symptoms. Hence currently treatments in VCFS target the specific deficits and symptoms presented by each child. It should be emphasized that VCFS is a very heterogeneous syndrome. Thus some children are only mildly affected cognitively and behaviorally while others can be severely affected. Most emotional and behavioral problems of VCFS should be treated using a multimodal approach. For some indications psychiatric medications are recommended but we believe psychiatric medications should always be accompanied by an appropriate psychosocial intervention. In addition, we believe that both parents and teachers should be involved in the treatment plan and its implementation.

### 1. Cognitive Behavioral Therapy (CBT)

Cognitive behavioral therapy (CBT) is considered the most effective psychological treatment for children and adolescents with anxiety disorders (James, Soler , & Weatherall, 2005). It is based on the premise that thoughts and feelings underlie behavior. To change behavior, cognitive behavioral therapists work to address and reduce distressing feelings and thoughts that may influence and/or change behavior. There are many different treatment strategies that focus on teaching the child and his parents how to master and overcome anxiety. Behavioral strategies are in general easier to implement and thus more effective than cognitive ones for children with VCFS. It is necessary for parents to be very involved in the treatment and that they will be well trained to manage the behavioral program.

### 2. Groups of Social Skills Training

Due to their social incompetence and immature social skills, children and adolescents with VCFS can benefit a great deal from participating in groups for social skills training. This kind of group intervention can serve as an intimate, secure, enabling environment for children who are shy, lack self-confidence, and are usually withdrawn from social interactions. The social skills training group psychotherapy affords the children and the therapists an opportunity to work on misperceptions and learn appropriate social behaviors in the "here and now." Analyzing the social interactions that occur during the meeting can help the children see the cause-effect relationship between their social behavior and the reactions of others (Lavoie, 2005).

### 3. Mentoring ("Big Brother") Program

In our Behavioral Neurogenetics Center in Israel we have been running a mentoring program for several years. In this mentoring program, young adults mentor children and adolescents with VCFS, for at least one year. The mentors, usually undergraduate psychology/social work students, meet the children in their homes for "one-on-one" interaction. The major goal of the program is to provide the children with a meaningful relationship that gives emotional support, encouragement, and advice. The mentors devote a considerable amount of the meetings to doing something fun with the child, allowing him to lead in doing things that give him a good feeling thus developing the child's sense of confidence. The mentor reveals interest in the child's inner world and his experiences and encourages the child to share what may be bothering him. As the relationship develops, the mentors serve as listening ears for the children, display empathy to their feelings, and provide support and advice. Once a bond has been formed and the child develops trust in the mentor, the groundwork is laid, and within this framework, structured therapeutic interventions, such as involving the mentor in the behavioral modification program of the child, are established in order to meet the specific difficulties of each child (DuBois, Holloway, Valentine, & Cooper, 2002).

### 4. Parent Guidance

Parent guidance is an essential component of the treatment in VCFS. The common issues that parents need guidance with are setting limits and encouraging their child's independence. Parents need assistance in learning how to set appropriate limits for their disabled child. Children tend to manifest oppositional behavior at home with their parents and siblings. Setting appropriate limits for the child is the most important component of dealing with the child's oppositional behavior. Setting appropriate limits is hard for the parents, as they often have to deal with their own guilt feelings and overidentification with the child's having to cope with multiple problems. Parents should be guided in how to be more firm and consistent with setting limits for the child and how to implement strategic use of praise, rewards, time outs, and contingency contracting (Bank, Marlowe, Reid, Patterson, & Weinrott, 1991).

Due to their disability, most children with VCFS are more dependent on their parents than typically developing children. Thus, parents of children with VCFS need to be more involved in various aspects of their daily life. They need to be active in making opportunities for social interactions for the child, and in encouraging him to widen his interests and helping him plan his leisure activities. However, and at the same time, it is important that parents encourage the child to develop maximum independence. The therapist and the parents should work together to define a gradual process in which the child will become less dependent in daily living skills, social functioning, and academics.

### 5. Psychiatric Medications

There is very little research on the safety and effectiveness of psychiatric medications in VCFS. Thus the guidelines that we suggest are based on studies of pediatric populations with similar psychiatric disorders. As VCFS is associated with a high rate of psychiatric disorders, we recommend that all children with VCFS be routinely evaluated by a child psychiatrist once every one to two years. During adolescence they should be evaluated more frequently because of the risk of evolution of psychotic disorders. It is important to initiate psychiatric treatment only following a thorough evaluation that will also include input from the school's teacher. A bad practice is to prescribe medication for "nonspecific behavioral problems" or "mood swings" instead of reaching the accurate psychiatric diagnosis first.

Since ADHD is the most common psychiatric disorder in VCFS the question of whether to prescribe stimulant medication is frequently raised. There are several concerns regarding the use of stimulants, such as Ritalin and Concerta, in subjects with VCFS. First, subjects with VCFS are at increased risk for the psychosis and depression that are possible side effects of these medications. Second, individuals with VCFS present with congenital cardiac anomalies that can increase their risk for cardiovascular side effects such as hypertension and tachycardia. There is only one open study that found that a low dose of Ritalin was beneficial for reducing the ADHD symptoms and safe in a one-month treatment of children with VCFS (Gothelf et al., 2003). Yet longer-term studies with placebo control groups are required to confirm the safety and effectiveness of stimulants and other medication treatments of ADHD in VCFS.

Symptoms of anxiety disorders, such as OCD, and symptoms of depressive disorders can be treated with serotonin-specific reuptake inhibitors such as Prozac. However, there is no data regarding the effect of these medications in VCFS. Our impression is that too many children and adolescents with VCFS in the United States receive mood-stabilizer medications such as Depakote. Our recommendation is that mood stabilizers only be prescribed for those VCFS subjects with manic episodes.

Another important and understudied therapeutic issue is the treatment of psychosis in VCFS. We recommend that all individuals with VCFS that manifest psychotic symptoms be evaluated by psychiatrists and prescribed antipsychotic medication. The findings that mild subthreshold psychotic symptoms tend to progress to a full-blown psychotic disorder suggest that it may be recommended to initiate antipsychotic treatment also in the milder cases of psychotic symptoms. This recommendation is supported by studies of schizophrenia in the general population that showed that prescribing antipsychotic medications early in the disease leads to a better outcome (Marshall et al., 2005). A study of five subjects with VCFS showed that metyrosine, a medication that lowers dopamine levels, has a beneficial effect on the psychotic symptoms of subjects with VCFS (Graf et al., 2001). However, metyrosine is not registered as an antipsychotic medication. There are no other studies about antipsychotics, commonly used for the treatment of schizophrenia in the general population, in VCFS individuals. Reports of case series suggest that, in general, subjects with VCFS are more vulnerable to side effects of antipsychotics and their psychotic symptoms have a lower rate of response compared to schizophrenia patients in the general population (Gothelf et al., 1999). Thus we recommend that psychiatrists treating subjects with VCFS will "start low and go slow" with antipsychotics and other psychiatric medications.

**Acknowledgement:** Supported in Part by Research Grant No. 5-FY06-590 from the March of Dimes Foundation and by the NARSAD Young Investigator Award.

# REFERENCES

Arnold, P. D., Siegel-Bartelt, .J, Cytrynbaum, C., Teshima, I., & Schachar, R. (2001) Velo-cardio-facial syndrome: Implications of microdeletion 22q11 for schizophrenia and mood disorders. *American Journal of Medical Genetics, 105,* 354–362.

Bank, L., Marlowe, J. H., Reid, J. B., Patterson, G. R., & Weinrott, M. R. (1991). A comparative evaluation of parent-training interventions for families of chronic delinquents. *Journal of Abnormal Child Psychology, 19,* 15–33.

Bassett, A. S., Chow, E. W., AbdelMalik, P., Gheorghiu, M., Husted, J., & Weksberg, R. (2003). The schizophrenia phenotype in 22q11 deletion syndrome. *American Journal of Psychiatry, 160,* 1580–1586.

Bassett, A. S., Hodgkinson, K., Chow, E. W., Correia, S., Scutt, L. E., & Weksberg, R. (1998). 22q11 deletion syndrome in adults with schizophrenia. *American Journal of Medical Genetics, 81,* 328–337.

Bielecki, J., & Swender, S. L. (2004). The assessment of social functioning in individuals with mental retardation: A review. *Behavior Modification, 28,* 694–708.

Burg, M., & Gothelf, D. (2003). *Self-concept in children with velocardiofacial syndrome.* In 9th Annual VCFES Conference, San Diego, CA.

Debbane, M., Glaser, B., Gex-Fabry, M., & Eliez, S. (2005). Temporal perception in velo-cardio-facial syndrome. *Neuropsychologia, 43,* 1754–1762.

DuBois, D. L., Holloway, B. E., Valentine, J. C., & Cooper, H. (2002). Effectiveness of mentoring programs for youth: A meta-analytic review. *American Journal of Community Psychology, 30,* 157–197.

Dykens, E. M .(2000). Psychopathology in children with intellectual disability. *Journal of Childhood Psychology and Psychiatry, 41,* 407–417.

Dykens, E. M., Leckman, J. F., & Cassidy, S. B. (1996). Obsessions and compulsions in Prader-Willi syndrome. *Journal of Childhood Psychology and Psychiatry, 37,* 995–1002.

Feinstein, C., Eliez, S., Blasey, C., & Reiss, A. L. (2002). Psychiatric disorders and behavioral problems in children with velocardiofacial syndrome: Usefulness as phenotypic indicators of schizophrenia risk. *Biological Psychiatry, 51,* 312–318.

Fine, S. E., Weissman, A., Gerdes, M., Pinto-Martin, J., Zackai, E. H., McDonald-McGinn, D. M., et al. (2005). Autism spectrum disorders and symptoms in children with molecularly confirmed 22q11.2 deletion syndrome. *Journal of Autism and Developmental Disorders, 35,* 461–470.

Geist, R., Grdisa, V., & Otley, A. (2003). Psychosocial issues in the child with chronic conditions. *Best Practice & Research. Clinical Gastroenterology, 17,* 141–152.

Gothelf, D., Eliez, S., Thompson, T., Hinard, C., Penniman, L., Feinstein C, et al. (2005). COMT genotype predicts longitudinal cognitive decline and psychosis in 22q11.2 deletion syndrome. *Nature and Neuroscience, 8,* 1500–1502.

Gothelf, D., Feinstein, C., Thompson, T., Van Stone, E., Gu, E., Penniman, L., et al. (in press). Risk factors for the emergence of psychotic disorders in adolescents with 22q11.2 deletion syndrome. *The American Journal of Psychiatry.*

Gothelf, D., Frisch, A., Munitz, H., Rockah, R., Laufer, N., Mozes, T., et al. (1999). Clinical characteristics of schizophrenia associated with velo-cardio-facial syndrome. *Schizophrenia Research, 35,* 105–112.

Gothelf, D., Gruber, R., Presburger, G., Dotan, I., Brand-Gothelf, A., Burg, M., et al. (2003). Methylphenidate treatment for attention-deficit/hyperactivity disorder in children and adolescents with velocardiofacial syndrome: An open-label study. *Journal of Clinical Psychiatry, 64,* 1163–1169.

Gothelf, D., Presburger, G., Zohar, A. H., Burg, M., Nahmani, A., Frydman, M., et al. (2004). Obsessive-compulsive disorder in patients with velocardiofacial (22q11 deletion) syndrome. *American Journal of Medical Genetics. Part B, Neuropsychiatric Genetics, 126,* 99–105.

Graf, W. D., Unis, A. S., Yates, C. M., Sulzbacher, S., Dinulos, M. B., Jack, R. M., et al. (2001). Catecholamines in patients with 22q11.2 deletion syndrome and the low-activity COMT polymorphism. *Neurology, 57,* 410–416.

James, A., Soler, A., & Weatherall, R. (2005). Cognitive behavioural therapy for anxiety disorders in children and adolescents. *Cochrane Database Systems Review,* (4), Article CD004690. Retrieved 2006 from http:www.cochrane.org/reviews/en/ab004690.html

Lavoie, R. (2005). *It's so much work to be your friend. Helping the child with learning disabilities find social success.* New York: Touchstone.

Marshall, M., Lewis, S., Lockwood, A., Drake, R., Jones, P., & Croudace, T. (2005). Association between duration of untreated psychosis and outcome in cohorts of first-episode patients: A systematic review. *Archives of General Psychiatry, 62,* 975–983.

Mervis, C. B., & Klein-Tasman, B. P. (2000). Williams syndrome: Cognition, personality, and adaptive behavior. *Mental Retardation and Developmental Disabilities Research Review, 6,* 148–158.

Murphy, K. C. (2002). Schizophrenia and velo-cardio-facial syndrome. *Lancet, 359,* 426–430.

Murphy, K. C., Jones, L. A., & Owen, M. J. (1999). High rates of schizophrenia in adults with velo-cardio-facial syndrome. *Archives of General Psychiatry, 56,* 940–945.

Papolos, D. F., Faedda, G. L., Veit, S., Goldberg, R., Morrow, B., Kucherlapati, R., et al. (1996). Bipolar spectrum disorders in patients diagnosed with velo-cardio-facial syndrome: Does a hemizygous deletion of chromosome 22q11 result in bipolar affective disorder? *American Journal of Psychiatry, 153,* 1541–1547.

Shprintzen, R. J. (2000). Velo-cardio-facial syndrome: A distinctive behavioral phenotype. *Mental Retardation and Developmental Disabilities Research Review, 6,* 142–147.

Shprintzen, R. J., Goldberg, R. B., Lewin, M. L., Sidoti, E. J., Berkman, M. D., Argamaso, R. V., et al. (1978). A new syndrome involving cleft palate, cardiac anomalies, typical facies, and learning disabilities: Velo-cardio-facial syndrome. *Cleft Palate Journal, 15,* 56–62.

Swillen, A., Devriendt, K., Ghesquiere, P., & Fryns, J. P. (2001). Children with a 22q11 deletion versus children with a speech-language impairment and learning disability: Behavior during primary school age. *Genetic Counseling, 12,* 309–317.

Swillen, A., Vandeputte, L., Cracco, J., Maes, B., Ghesquiere, P., Devriendt, K., et al. (1999). Neuropsychological, learning and psychosocial profile of primary school aged children with the velo-cardio-facial syndrome (22q11 deletion): Evidence for a nonverbal learning disability? *Child Neuropsychology, 5,* 230–241.

Turner, T. H. (1989). Schizophrenia and mental handicap: An historical review, with implications for further research. *Psychological Medicine, 19,* 301–314.

Wing, L., & Gould, J. (1979). Severe impairments of social interaction and associated abnormalities in children: Epidemiology and classification. *Journal of Autism and Developmental Disorders, 9,* 11–29.

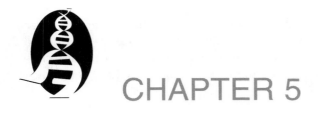

# CHAPTER 5

# Communication in Velo-Cardio-Facial Syndrome

## KAREN GOLDING-KUSHNER, PhD

*V*erbal communication includes both language and speech. It has been reported that a high percentage of children with VCFS have problems affecting both speech and language. Communication development in children with VCFS was reviewed by Golding-Kushner (2005, p. 195). She summarized,

> Children with VCFS are at very high risk for communicative impairment. Further, the communication skills of children with VCFS may be syndrome-specific and are typically characterized by severe VPI, hypernasality and a glottal stop articulation disorder. Onset of language is typically delayed with receptive language developing more rapidly than expressive and with severe deficits in early vocabulary acquisition and speech sound production. Speech and expressive language show rapid improvement between age 3 and 4 years but specific language impairment persists and, even as language continues to improve, working memory, reasoning, abstract thinking, and social language present challenges. Individuals with VCFS respond well to direct teaching in therapy and academics, but intensive and frequent repetition is necessary for mastery and application of new skills and concepts. The combination of aggressive articulation therapy and surgical correction of VPI results in normal speech and resonance. Language therapy and a need for academic support typically continue throughout the school years.

This chapter will explain language and speech, summarize the nature of the communication disorders most common in VCFS and how to assess them, and describe effective treatment. It will also address issues related to the child, clinician, and parents that occur when treatment occurs in the school setting.

## SPEECH AND LANGUAGE IN VCFS

*Speech* refers to the mechanical aspects of verbal communication: the sound of the voice, resonance, articulation, and fluency. *Language* refers to the symbolic aspect of communication.

## SPEECH

### Voice

Voice refers to the sound produced by the larynx (voice box) and is heard throughout speech (except during whispering). Three aspects of voice are quality, volume, and pitch.

**Quality.** Vocal fold vibration occurs along the length of the vocal folds and is normally smooth and symmetric. During the closed phase of the vibratory cycle, closure between the two vocal folds should be smooth and complete. Any abnormality in the structure of one or both folds, or in their ability to move together and vibrate in a synchronous and symmetric manner, may result in excess airflow through the glottis, or space between the vocal folds. This excess flow of air through the glottis caused by incomplete glottal closure is perceived as breathiness or, when more extreme, hoarseness. Vocal fold anomalies such as unilateral vocal fold paresis, asymmetry in size of the vocal folds, and laryngeal web have been reported in more than 35% of children with VCFS (Chegar, Tatum, Marrinan, & Shprintzen, 2006). These anomalies may result in a hoarse vocal quality. Hoarseness has also been reported in children with velopharyngeal insufficiency (VPI), especially if VPI is mild. It has been hypothesized that this may be a result of the speaker's attempt to increase respiratory pressure at the level of the larynx to compensate for loss of air pressure through the velopharynx. Thus, some hoarseness among children with VCFS may be related to VPI. By far, the most common cause of hoarseness in school-aged children is vocal misuse or vocal abuse, resulting in excessive laryngeal tension and leading to vocal fold edema or even vocal fold nodules. Examples of vocal abuse are singing at a pitch that is too high or too low for that child's larynx, yelling, imitating car and animal sounds, and chronic coughing or throat clearing. Children with VCFS may experience hoarseness due to these same vocal abuses.

**Volume.** Volume, or vocal loudness, is controlled by respiratory flow from the lungs. When airflow from the lungs is increased, volume is louder. Children with VCFS often speak with a soft, quiet voice. In VCFS, this is not typically caused by decreased lung capacity or an actual deficiency in respiratory ability. Reduced volume (loudness) is more likely to be related to conductive hearing loss, velopharyngeal insufficiency resulting in loss of air pressure, vocal fold anomalies preventing adequate vocal fold closure to generate a strong sound signal, or personality. Some speakers may intentionally speak softly in an attempt to reduce nasal emission or hypernasality (Peterson-Falzone, Trost-Cardamone, Karnell, & Hardin-Jones, 2001).

**Pitch.** Pitch is the perception of the frequency of vibration of the vocal folds and is related to their length and thickness. High vocal pitch has been reported to be common in children with VCFS and may be caused by a laryngeal web, which effectively shortens the vibrating segments of the fold, or laryngeal immaturity.

### Treatment of Voice Problems

Speech therapy to ameliorate a voice problem should never be attempted until the larynx and velopharynx have been examined to identify any anatomic or physiologic pathology causing the problem. Some issues can be resolved therapeutically but others cannot, and therapy should not be implemented to correct disorders of voice unless the child has had a thorough examination by an otolaryngologist (ENT physician), and the ENT and speech-language pathologist (SLP) have discussed the situation. Treatment of hoarseness related to vocal abuse may include vocal counseling to establish awareness of the vocal behaviors that must be curtailed. Respiratory exercises that increase control of respiratory support may be useful in increasing volume. There are also exercises to change pitch, but they should never be applied if the perceived elevated pitch is the appropriate pitch for the size of the vocal folds, even if it is an inappropriate pitch for age, because that could cause further vocal abuse and vocal fold damage. Detailed suggestions for voice therapy may be found in several standard speech pathology textbooks including Boone, McFarlane, & Von Berg, 2004, and Rubin, Sataloff, & Korovin, 2006.

### Resonance

Resonance is a characteristic imposed on the speech signal as the sound from the larynx passes through the vocal tract. At the top of the vocal tract is the opening between the oropharynx (the part of the throat behind the mouth) and the nasopharynx (the top of the throat behind the nasal cavity). This opening is known as the velopharyngeal orifice. During normal speech, the velopharyngeal (VP) mechanism opens and closes, depending on the speech sounds being produced. This opening and closing is mediated by the movements of the soft palate (velum) and the pharyngeal walls. The sounds *m, n,* and *ng* are nasal, meaning that air must exit through the nose during production of those sounds. Velopharyngeal closure occurs over time, as well as over space, so there is some velopharyngeal opening during production of the sounds immediately preceding and following the nasal consonant. When VP opening is constricted or occurs for too short a duration, resonance is perceived as hyponasal, or denasal. This is the way one sounds when congested with a cold. The opposite, velopharyngeal insufficiency (VPI), results when complete velopharyngeal closure does not occur during production of non-nasal sounds. The terms velopharyngeal inadequacy and velopharyngeal incompetence are sometimes used to describe VPI of different etiology, but all may be referred to as VPI, and that generic designation will be used throughout this chapter for simplicity.

VPI is one of the most common characteristics of the speech of children with VCFS. The high frequency of VPI is related to several underlying anatomic features. Among them are cleft palate, submucous cleft palate and occult submucous cleft palate, an obtuse cranial base angle resulting in increased pharyngeal depth, a small adenoid, and thin and abnormal pharyngeal muscle tissue. This is described in more detail in Golding-Kushner (1991, 2001, 2005).

A high percentage of children with VCFS have hypertrophied tonsils resulting in a muffling of the oral resonance, sometimes referred to as "potato-in-the-mouth" or "marshmallow-in-the-mouth" resonance. The speaker sounds as if he or she tried to swallow marshmallows that became lodged in the back of the mouth. In this situation, the tonsils do not typically appear to be infected (until analyzed after removal), and may not contribute to a high frequency of strep infections, leading many physicians to dismiss their size as insignificant. However, they may cause the abnormal oral resonance just described and may contribute to tongue fronting leading to a pattern of articulation errors in which the tongue is forward and even protruding. Non-speech sequelae often include feeding problems such as preferences for soft foods and slow, picky eating habits, coughing (Shprintzen, 2005), and airway obstruction during sleep. Therefore, the potential significance of their size should not be overlooked. Tonsil size may appear different when examined orally and endoscopically. The endoscopic view is a more accurate representation of the size and postion of the tonsils relative to the airway (Traquina, Golding-Kushner, and Shprintzen, 1990).

### *Articulation*

Articulation refers to the actual production of speech sounds, or pronunciation. The most common articulation problems encountered in VCFS are articulation delay, phonological disorder, and compensatory speech disorders, sometimes called "cleft palate speech."

**Articulation Delay.** Articulation is described as delayed when a child begins to produce a sound at a later age than the age at which most children produce the same sound, or when he or she substitutes an early developing sound for a later developing sound. Examples are substitution of *th* for *s* and *w* for *r*. This type of articulation problem is common among typically-developing children and tends to respond easily to traditional articulation therapy.

**Phonological Disorder.** In a phonological disorder, errors affect large classes of sounds. Acceptable sounds are substituted and rearranged within words and phrases in an unacceptable but predictable manner, although the errors may *seem* inconsistent without in-depth analysis. For example, a child may substitute "**c**ook" for "**t**ook" but produce a perfectly correct /t/ in the word "tea." For this child, speech production may be governed by a rule that says, "If there is a back sound in the word, produce all consonants as back sounds; if not, produce the /t/." Like articulation delay, this type of problem is also common among typically developing children.

There are many approaches to correcting phonological disorders, most of which include a significant component referred to as "auditory bombardment." In this approach, the clinician presents extensive examples of correct production of the patterns that have not developed and the child is expected to hear enough examples to extract the correct rule (such as, "It's okay to have a back consonant such as *k* and a front consonant such as *t* in the same word.") and, in turn, apply it to his or her own speech production. This approach is not particularly effective with children with VCFS because they typically do not learn well using exploration techniques. Rather, as Landsman explained (2004, 2006, Chapter 10 in this book), they learn best using direct instructional approaches.

Another common approach to phonological disorders is the cycles approach (Hodson & Paden, 1991). In this approach, sounds produced according to a particular rule are targeted for a specified period of time, after which a new rule is stimulated, regardless of mastery of production of the first set of sounds. This would not be consistent with our understanding of how children with VCFS learn and would not, therefore, be a good choice for a treatment approach. Later in this chapter, the general therapy principles that have proven effective in correcting articulation delay and phonological patterns of errors will be discussed.

**"Cleft Palate" Speech.** Certain patterns of articulation errors are strongly associated with cleft palate and VPI and rarely occur in speakers who have good velopharyngeal closure. Therefore, these errors have come to be referred to as "cleft palate speech," even though the speaker may not have a cleft palate. This is the most frequently occurring speech disorder in children with VCFS. It was explained in the previous section why VPI is so common in this population. It follows that this is the most common articulation disorder. This type of speech disorder is not "outgrown" and may seem resistant to therapy. This pattern of speech includes two categories of errors: *obligatory errors* and *compensatory errors*.

*Obligatory Errors:* As suggested by the name, obligatory errors are directly caused by an anatomic or physiological anomaly and cannot be avoided. Examples are nasal emission of air during speech and consequent loss of normal intraoral air pressure during speech because of VPI. Before attempting to correct these errors using speech therapy, the velopharyngeal mechanism must be visualized using a direct technique such as nasopharyngoscopy or multiview videofluoroscopy to determine if the child ever achieves complete velopharyngeal closure during speech. If not, as is the case with most children with VCFS, the errors are obligatory and cannot be corrected using speech therapy. They will resolve without therapy following physical management of VPI.

*Compensatory errors:* This category of errors includes mistakes that may be an attempt to compensate for loss of air pressure through the velopharyngeal valve by producing the sound at a level closer to the larynx, the source of air pressure. Examples are glottal stops, pharyngeal fricatives, nasal snorting, or velar fricative. These are the most common errors among children with VCFS and, although caused by VPI, are learned, not obligatory, and must be treated using speech therapy. These errors seem to be the most resistant to therapy but do respond well to the general principles and some special techniques to be described. These errors are, unfortunately, often misdiagnosed as consonant omissions or even as apraxia or dyspraxia because there is typically a lack of tongue and lip movement during speech attempts. However, this speech disorder is very different from apraxia.

Glottal stops occur when the vocal folds are used to create a "stop" sound at the level of the larynx. This replaces use of the lips or tongue to produce a sound in the mouth. The lip or tongue movement is sometimes coproduced with a glottal stop, but is usually omitted. Pharyngeal fricatives are generally produced as substitutions for fricative and some sibilant sounds (*f, v, th, s, z, sh*) and also as substitutions for affricates *ch* and *j*. Like glottal stops, they maintain the manner of production, that is, the attempt to produce a continuous stream of air through a constriction, but are produced closer to the larynx than normal. Nasal snorting occurs when air is forcibly emitted through the nares instead of through the mouth. This is different from nasal emission, which is a passive leak of air through the nose. Pinching the nares during a nasal snort results in an absence of sound, whereas pinching the nares during nasal emission results in a correctly articulated sound.

Speech intelligibility is most severely compromised in children with compensatory articulation errors because the sounds being produced are atypical and because there is a lack of differentiation among sounds. As stated above, compensatory errors can only be corrected using speech therapy. Surgery to eliminate VPI does not change compensatory patterns, although occasionally, the response to therapy is enhanced if VPI is eliminated first. In children with cleft palate who do not have VCFS, velopharyngeal closure is sometimes improved when compensatory errors are eliminated (Golding-Kushner, 1980, 1995, 2001). Therefore, it has been recommended that therapy precede surgery to treat VPI. However, this has not typically been observed in children with VCFS. Therefore the sequence of therapy and surgery in VCFS may not be critical.

### Fluency

Stuttering has not been reported as a problem in children with VCFS. It could certainly occur, but would not be expected to occur more frequently than in the general population and is not a feature of the syndrome.

## LANGUAGE

*Language* refers to the symbolic aspect of communication and includes receptive function, or comprehension, and an expressive function. Language may also be described in terms of its form, content, and use. In this paradigm, language *form* refers to the syntactic and morphologic aspects of the message. Language *content* refers to the meaning of language, or the concepts understood and expressed. The third aspect, language *use*, is the pragmatic feature of communication. This is the social aspect of language and one that is frequently difficult for children with VCFS. Pragmatics includes application of language to take the listener's needs into account in formulating a statement, understanding sarcasm and subtle language messages, staying on a topic during conversation, and using language for a variety of purposes, such as to request information, to share information, to initiate contact, to avoid confrontation, and so on.

## SPEECH AND LANGUAGE THERAPY AT SCHOOL

The majority of children with language, learning, and speech problems receive therapeutic intervention at school. In order to be eligible to receive services at school, criteria related to thresholds of severity must be met. In addition, the communication disorder must have some educational impact for the student to be eligible, even if severity criteria are met.

### Preschool: Ages 3 to 5 Years

Preschool children with VCFS typically have significant articulation deficits that qualify them for therapy at school. However, they may test well on certain aspects of language function so the test battery must be selected carefully to identify areas of need. A comprehensive language evaluation should be performed even if language skills seem intact superficially because of the high risk for language and learning disorders among children with VCFS. The assessment battery should include a test that taps into a broad range of language skills. Examples of tests that cover a broad range of receptive and expressive language skills for children in this age range are the Clinical Evaluation of Language Functions-Preschool (CELF-P) and the Preschool Language Scale-4 (PLS-4). When results of the general tests are reviewed, additional testing may be done to obtain more detailed information on the specific aspects of language identified as weak. Examples of these more focused tests are the Receptive- and Expressive-One-Word-Picture Vocabulary Tests (ROWPVT and EOWPVT). Another sensitive test of receptive language, and a test of auditory memory, is the Token Test for Children. This test includes five sections and requires the child to follow directions involving manipulation of tokens of two sizes, two shapes, and five colors. The directions are increasingly complex and contain two to six critical elements. The Preschool Language Assessment Instrument-2 (PLAI) identifies language and communication difficulties that might interfere with classroom performance. The test looks at how effectively a child integrates cognitive, linguistic, and pragmatic components to deal with the adult-child conversations. It is also important to obtain a spontaneous speech sample for analysis. The tests listed are among the more commonly used, but the list is by no means exhaustive and includes only a few of the hundreds of tests available.

## School: Ages 5 to 21

Most children with 22q11.2 deletion require some type of speech therapy, language therapy, or both during their school years. It is hoped that by age 5, the articulation errors will be corrected. However, this is often still an area of therapeutic need. The language deficits may become more apparent during the middle-elementary years (grade three or four) because it is at that time that language is used for learning and concepts are more abstract. Rote and concrete skills may be relatively strong, so it is, again, important to select a test battery that looks at a wide range of skills. In most states in the United States, in order to qualify for language therapy at school, it is necessary to obtain a Standard Score more that 1.5 standard deviations below the mean on two tests of language. If the student has low scores on several subtests, but the overall language score is better than 1.5 standard deviations below the mean, the student will not qualify. Because he or she may have strong skills in certain areas that, on average, counterbalance the low scores in other areas, testing beyond the general tests is often necessary. In middle school and high school, it is especially important to test higher order skills involved in inferential thinking and similar abstract processes.

# THERAPY AT SCHOOL

School-based speech-language pathologists in schools face many challenges. These include attitudes, training, scheduling, and communication.

Speech and language therapy services are available privately, in clinics, and in hospitals. In these settings, parental participation in the process and specific parent training to work with children at home is easily accomplished. Sessions are almost always individual. The child does not have to be pulled out of the classroom resulting in a missed lesson, or in being singled out in front of classmates. In contrast, therapy at school is not always consistent, through no fault of the speech specialist. Students miss speech when there is a class trip, when there is a special assembly, or when there is some other special program in the classroom, such as a party or guest. Why, then, schedule therapy at school, where there are so many obvious disadvantages? There are distinct advantages. Sessions can be scheduled several times a week without concern about interfering with other outside activities and without concern about transportation to a hospital or clinic. The child, as long as he or she is in school, is available for the session. Therapy goals can, and, in some states by law, must, be integrated with the general classroom curriculum. Finally, therapy at school is free of charge to the family, which can be a major financial benefit when considered over a long period of time. The fact is, in the United States, most children do receive their speech and language therapy at school.

Unfortunately, very few graduate training programs in speech pathology require students to take a course in cleft palate or craniofacial syndromes. Students at one university refused to take the course in cleft palate and syndromes because they intended to work in schools and believed that children with cleft palate or related syndromes would not be part of their caseload. This misguided attitude kept them from taking the very course(s) that would give them proper training to meet the needs of children with VCFS. This is an issue currently being addressed by the American Cleft Palate Craniofacial Association, but it is the American Speech-Language-Hearing Association that sets standards for graduate training programs and the requirement for a course in a medically-based disorder class is usually met with a course in aphasia, not cleft palate. This means that, at least at this time, most speech pathologists working in schools have little, if any, training in syndromes, and may not be at all familiar with velo-cardio-facial syndrome. Fortunately, there are many opportunities for continuing education, and participating in continuing education is required by many states to maintain credentials to work in schools, and by the American Speech-Language-Hearing Association.

## Qualifying for Services

In order to be eligible for speech and language services at school, a child must meet certain criteria that are generally based on test scores. In most states, it is total test scores that are used, not scores on subtests. Therefore, it is important for the speech pathologist doing the testing to know the areas of weakness and select tests accordingly. The case study presented later in this chapter describes Abby, a student who was receiving articulation therapy, and how her evaluation had to be supplemented for her to qualify to receive language therapy. When the "standard" battery of tests, administered in a one and a half-hour test session, was used, she did not qualify. The child study team was satisfied with the outcome, concluded that she did not need to be classified, said she was not eligible for language therapy, and hoped the speech pathologist would agree and not pursue the suspected need for language intervention. However, she did not. She looked at the subtests that showed weaknesses and administered tests specifically to target those skills. This required two additional hours of testing. However, creative testing by the SLP resulted in Abby's qualifying for both speech *and* language services. The child study team was not very happy with the clinician who did the evaluation, because they did not want the therapist to use so much testing time on one student, and did not want the student to consume more of the therapist's treatment time and resources.

There certainly are children who do have deficits in speech, language, or both who need therapy but really do *not* qualify for services at school, even with the most extensive testing. This is because they may have several areas of borderline or low skill, but not "low enough." Parents must understand that does not mean therapy is not needed or that it would not be beneficial. It means only that the child does not qualify to receive those services at taxpayer expense during the school day, and treatment should be sought in another venue.

## INDIVIDUALIZED EDUCATIONAL PLANS (IEPs)

Once it is determined that a child is eligible to receive speech and language therapy at school, an IEP must be developed. The IEP includes a statement of the problem, an academic impact statement, a list of long-term goals to be addressed that school year, and a list of related objectives, which are short-term goals that must be achieved in order to accomplish the long-term goal. The IEP also includes a list of any accommodations that may be necessary based on the communication problem, and a list of procedures that will be implemented to achieve the goals and objectives. Finally, the IEP states how progress will be measured, and the manner and frequency with which parents will be informed of progress.

Speech pathologists may have as many as 80 students on their caseload. Because of the inordinate amount of time it would take to write a detailed IEP on each student, most school districts have computerized templates that are used and clinicians fill in codes to represent goals and objectives listed in a reference book. They select criterion levels for reaching goals from a drop-down list. There is also a general list from which to choose the way in which the goals will be measured. This list includes choices such as "Therapist generated materials," or "Observation of Teacher." Other methods can be written in by the therapist, but the choices are all vague. In fact, they are often deliberately left vague in order to give the therapist some latitude. Parents should insist that the goals and objectives included in the IEP are specific to their child's needs, even if the clinician must write the goals because the reference book does not include the exact objective that would be appropriate.

IEPs in some districts include a statement of procedures that will be used, but this is also generally kept extremely vague, so that the parents may, in fact, have no idea of the procedures to be used, especially with regard to the articulation deficits. The parents of a child with VCFS should insist on detail, to be sure inappropriate procedures are not being used. Procedures for articulation therapy should include imitation of sounds in syllables, words, and phrases, drill, and so on. They should not include exercises to increase the strength or range of motion of the articulators, massage, blowing, sucking, or other nonspeech tasks. These procedures do not improve speech production, voice, or resonance (Powers & Starr, 1974; Christensen & Hanson, 1981; Ruscello, 1982; Starr, 1990; Van Demark & Hardin, 1990; Peterson-Falzone et al., 2006).

The IEP also lists the model, or method through which services will be provided, the number of times per week therapy will be scheduled, and a statement as to whether therapy will be provided individually or in groups. Because they learn best with repetition and rehearsal, therapy for children with VCFS should occur at least three times per week, and this should be supplemented by a daily home program.

## Model

Traditionally, services in schools were provided using a pull-out model, in which students are pulled out of the classroom to go to a speech session in another room with the speech specialist. This remains the most common method of service delivery in schools and, for most children with VCFS, is the most effective model. Students are pulled out individually or, more commonly, in groups ranging in size from two to five children. Clinicians make an effort to group students according to the nature of their therapy needs but the grouping is also influenced by other factors such as class schedule, schedule of other services being received by the student, and grade placement. As a result, students in a group may have needs that are similar or, in some cases, quite diverse.

Another model of service delivery is a push-in model, in which the speech specialist goes into the classroom and provides services to one or several students in the class while the teacher is teaching a lesson. This could prove distracting for children with VCFS, who may have difficulty screening out irrelevant stimuli and concentrating on a specific task.

In a collaborative model, the speech specialist and classroom teacher consult about the curriculum and how speech/language goals can be met while working through the curriculum in the classroom.

The maximum size of groups for pull-out and push-in models is specified by each state and, in New Jersey, for example, can be as large as five students. Most districts encourage therapists to arrange large groups to save money, and, unless otherwise specified, the default group size will be the largest allowed by law. Children with VCFS learn well in a one-to-one situation, so individual therapy is beneficial, especially for speech therapy. For language therapy or for speech therapy when the target is mastery of sounds in dialogue, a group of two may be beneficial *if* the two students have similar needs.

In some IEP templates there is not a place to specify group size. However, it can be written in by the speech pathologist. It may be up to the parents, acting as advocates on behalf of their child, to be sure the recommendation for the most appropriate group size is specified. Parents should insist that group size be specified in writing. Child study teams must sometimes be reminded that the "I" in "IEP" stands for "Individualized"! Parents should also check in with the speech pathologist periodically to be sure the group size has not been modified to accommodate another child's change in schedule or a therapist's change in schedule.

## Procedures

Certain things we know about how children with VCFS tend to learn must be applied to speech therapy. Specifically, we know that they learn best using direct teaching methods; "discovery" methods of learning are not as effective. Also, we know that they require a lot of repetition to learn. For speech therapy, then, methods that provide both direct instruction and multiple opportunities for rehearsal of the new skill are best. Behavior modification is a very effective tool for both articulation and language therapy. Verbal praise is one form of positive reinforcement, but most children tire of that alone and maintain motivation and focus more consistently when some other tangible reward is earned. Positive reinforcement should be provided after correct responses on a consistent schedule, and that schedule should be modified according to the student's level of mastery. When learning a new skill, reinforcement might be provided after every correct response. As mastery increases, it might be provided after every three or five correct responses. The reinforcer must be something valued by the student, such as a sticker on a chart, a piece to a puzzle, a turn at a game, and so on. However, it should not be something that is distracting that would interfere with achieving the goal of the session. If it is not earned, it should be withheld, or it loses value. This may be frustrating for some children, but it is part of behavior modification.

## Direct Instruction

### Articulation Therapy

Tell the child exactly how to produce the target sound. State where to place the articulators and specify that air should be directed through the mouth and not the nose. A drill approach is most effective with children with VCFS. Clinicians may provide a variety of sources of support for sound production, including auditory cues (producing the model), verbal instructions, visual cues (mirror, modeling), tactile cues (such as feeling a puff of air produced during /h/ on the hand), graphic cues, and even manual assistance (holding the lips closed to help the child produce /m, p, b/). Sounds should be introduced in a logical sequence, and the child should demonstrate mastery at simple levels of production, such as syllables or words, before working on more advanced levels of production. When eliminating glottal stops, whispering is useful because it creates a physiologic conflict with production of a glottal stop. Nasal occlusion is useful in the elimination of nasal snorting because it prevents airflow through the nose and teaches oral air escape instead. A variety of procedures and more detail about the techniques listed here are described in Golding-Kushner, 2001.

### Home Practice

Home practice is an essential component of the speech therapy program, especially for articulation therapy. Without *daily* practice, the skills will not be integrated into conversational speech for a protracted period of time, if at all. Therefore, an important role of the school SLP is to provide a daily home program of practice. This practice cannot occur without the assistance of an adult "speech helper" at home, usually a parent. The speech helper cannot do this effectively without detailed instructions and training. This presents a challenge to school SLPs, most of whom tend to see parents infrequently, and then only at child study team meetings or end-of-year reviews, and who are unaccustomed to working closely with parents on a daily or weekly basis. The training could be useful to parents of children with other articulation disorders as well, so the clinician may want to schedule a group training session in the evening at the beginning of the school year for several parents at once. During that session, the general principles of therapy can be explained and specific techniques for positive reinforcement can be taught. The home practice should trail therapy by one level, so anything being done at home is reinforcing and strengthening new skills, not introducing them. The specific target words to be practiced at home should be written in the speech book, or pictures of those words should be provided, so that the selection of target words is in the hands of the clinician, not the speech helper. This ensures that the words practiced are appropriate in terms of phonetic content (that is, which sounds are in the word) and phonetic complexity (the number of syllables and sequence of sounds in the word). Practice sessions at home should take no more than 5 or 10 minutes at a time, and home practice should occur at least twice a day. This rarely places an undue burden on parents or children, who may have significant amounts of homework in other areas. It is important that students and parents understand that there are no "free passes" for speech home practice. If children are speaking at all during a particular day, they are practicing their errors; they do not get a "vacation" from practicing the correct production for a few minutes. To the extent possible (that is, to the extent that they fit the phonetic criteria), target words should come from the curriculum, and may be taken from any subject, even math (e.g., *two, ten* when working on /t/). Instructions sent home should be very specific and very easy to follow. For example, the clinician might write,

> Say each word and tell Sara to repeat it after you. Tell her to "make windy lips." After she repeats the word, tell her "Good, that was windy," or, if she made an error, say, "You used your lips but forgot the wind. Try again." Then say the word again for her to repeat and exaggerate the element that was incorrect in her production. Do this until she produces each word on the list correctly five times. If she makes an error, it does not count toward the five.

To save time, a worksheet can be prepared in advance and completed during the session, when a decision can be made as to the target words and level of practice that should follow (Figure 5–1).

## STORY OF ABBY AND QUALIFYING TESTS

Although she had the 22q11.2 microdeletion, Abby's profile was not typical of students with VCFS. She had no palatal abnormality, and voice was within normal limits. Resonance was hypernasal. She had only recently been diagnosed with the 22q11.2 microdeletion. She was in a regular class with support from her classroom teacher for certain subjects and her parents had her tutored in several subjects outside of school to help her keep up with her class. However, she had never been evaluated by the child study team and was not classified. Her case is included because it illustrates the difficulty that the therapist encountered in qualifying her for language therapy, and how it was accomplished.

HOMEWORK FOR *Jimmy* **SPEECH LANGUAGE** THERAPY          DATE 9/22/06

We are practicing *imitating the sound "hhhhh" at the beginning of syllables*
Please   _X_ repeat after your speech helper
          ___read each syllable/word
          ___say the phrase _____ for each word
          ___make up a sentence for each word
          ___other: _____

         Do this _10_ times CORRECTLY each day for each *word.* If you make a mistake, it does
not count. Try again. **Start the day on which you had therapy: things are fresh in your mind and
success is more likely!!!!** *Practice 5 of the words in the morning or right after
school and the other 5 words before bed time so there are two very short
practice sessions each day. (Pick two other times if those are not
convenient for your family.)*

Hints for the speech helper:  Remind your child to:
*Say the word and have Jimmy repeat after you. Tell him, "Open your
mouth and make big wind." When it is correct, say, "Good wind!" If he
forgets the wind say, "You forgot the wind. Make it windy" and say the
word again. Exaggerate the "h." Hold your palm in front of his mouth
to be sure you can also feel the wind. Let him feel it also.*

Words (please check above if child is to REPEAT after you or SAY it without a model)
1. *hay*          4. *ho* ☐          7. *ham*                    10. *hem*
2. *he*           5. *who*           8. *him*
3. *hi*           6. *home*          9. *hum*

Sign on the line for that day when the practice session is over. **If you miss a day, skip that line so
we know which days your child REALLY practiced.  You cannot practice on Wednesday for
Tuesday! If the day is gone, it's gone.** If you run out of lines, ADD MORE and write the day/date.
Please write any comments about difficulty or success that will help me plan the next therapy session
and the next homework.

| Day/Date | Signature | Comments |
|---|---|---|
| *Fri 9/22* | _____ | _____ |
| *Sat 9/23* | _____ | _____ |
| *Sun 9/24* | _____ | _____ |
| *Mon 9/25* | _____ | _____ |

*See you Monday! Remember to bring your speech book!*
IF YOU RUN OUT OF SPACES, ADD MORE LINES AND DATES ON THE BACK OF THIS SHEET OR ON
ANOTHER PAPER AND **KEEP PRACTICING THE SAME** HOMEWORK UNTIL I GIVE YOU A NEW PAPER!!!!

**FIGURE 5–1.** Homework worksheet used at school for articulation therapy homework. Used with permission of Karen Golding-Kushner.

## Background

Abby, a 10–year, 4-month old girl in fourth grade, received speech therapy at school to improve production of /s/. She had recently begun working on production of /r/. The child study team met with Abby's parents for her annual review, as mandated by law. Her parents expressed concern about persistent difficulty with reading and subjects in which instruction relied heavily on reading, such as social studies. The teacher reported that she had seen good progress in reading with extra support Abby received in and out of class, but stated that Abby had persistent difficulty with reading and spelling. Abby's mother also asked about her perception that there were discrepancies in language skills in previous reports and requested additional testing in that area. Because of concern about auditory processing skills, the school nurse, who had screened Abby's hearing and vision earlier in the school year, repeated the hearing test and Abby passed the screening at 20 dB in both ears, indicating normal peripheral hearing. Abby was reevaluated to determine continued eligibility for speech therapy and to determine if she had a need for language therapy.

## Observation

Abby maintained attention to task and demonstrated excellent focus for extended testing periods (one to one and a half hours with short breaks).

## Basis for Evaluation

Observation

Oral peripheral examination

The Goldman-Fristoe Test of Articulation-2

Receptive One-Word Picture Vocabulary Test-Revised

Expressive One-Word Picture Vocabulary Test-Revised

The Test of Auditory Processing Skills (TAPS-3)

The Token Test for Children

The Phonological Awareness Test

The Word-R Test

## Evaluation Results

### *Speech*

**Oral Peripheral Examination.** An examination of the articulators revealed normal structure. The left ear was slightly anterior to the right ear, but symmetry was otherwise good and examination was unremarkable. Dentition was characterized by mild lateral crossbites but that did not interfere with articulation. The palate was normal in appearance and to palpation, nasal emission was positive on a mirror test. There was no evidence of apraxia, dysarthria, or oral-motor dysfunction.

**Voice.** Vocal pitch, volume, and quality were within normal limits for Abby's age and gender.

**Resonance.** Resonance was moderately hypernasal. Oral resonance was normal.

**Fluency.** Rate and fluency were within normal limits.

### Articulation

*Goldman-Fristoe Test of Articulation-2.* The Goldman-Fristoe Test of Articulation-2 was administered to supplement analysis of a speech sample. On the Sounds-in-Words subtest, Abby's raw score of 23 errors corresponded to an age equivalent of 3 years, 4 months. On this test, a standard score between 85 and 115 is considered average. Abby's standard score was 46 (below the first percentile), indicating significantly below average articulation skills. Her speech pattern while naming pictures with single words was consistent with her speech on the Sounds-in-Sentences subtest and during conversation. She had worked on /s/ and /s/ blends in therapy and there were no errors on that sound, either in words or in conversation, indicating complete mastery. She also worked on /z/, which was produced correctly most of the time but sometimes produced as /s/. Other errors included production of /n, t, d, l/ with interdental tongue tip placement, resulting in a visual speech error, and substitution of w/r, resulting in speech distortion. She also inserted /f/ before final -*th*, as in "bafth" for "bath." Speech was intelligible most of the time, although noticeably in error. Stimulability for correct production of error sounds was fair.

### *Language*

### Receptive One-Word Picture Vocabulary Test (ROWPVT)

| | |
|---|---|
| Raw Score: | 92 |
| Standard Score: | 90 (Mean = 100 +/− 15) |
| Percentile Rank: | 25 |
| Age Equivalent: | 8–9 |

The ROWPVT assessed comprehension of single words. The student is presented three pictures and points to the one named or described. Abby's responses were thoughtful and deliberate, and her score was in the average range.

## Expressive One-Word Picture Vocabulary Test-R (EOWTPVT-R)

Raw Score:            76

Standard Score:    80 (Mean = 100 +/– 15)

Percentile Rank:    9

Age Equivalent:    7–4

The Expressive One-Word Picture Vocabulary Test-R assessed ability to retrieve single words to name pictures. Abby's score was below average. She had difficulty with word retrieval and made semantic (meaning) and phonetic (sound) errors. She generally described the objects correctly, indicating that she knew their identity and function, but could not name them. At times, she successfully cued herself by stating function and then arrived at the correct name. For example, for "cactus," she said, "It's a plant—in the desert—it's uh—oh (delayed a few seconds)—a cactus." When shown a pineapple, she said, "A fruit—I know it but I can't think of it." For compass she said, "It's a toy that tells you what direction to go." For windmill she said, "I'm not sure— oh, a wind blower." She said "lettuce" for celery, "nail file" for tweezers, and "wheel barrier" for wheelbarrow. She called a graph "score keeper" and for boomerang said, "I know it, oh, it's like that thing that you throw it and it come right backs to you."

The difference in scores between the RWOPVT and EOWPVT was significant but not meaningful because, according to the test publisher, differences of that magnitude are common.

**The Test of Auditory Processing Skills (TAPS-3).** This test was administered because of concern about Abby's auditory processing skills, which can affect reading and writing. This test includes nine subtests, summarized on the chart below.

| Subtest | Raw Score | Scaled Score (Mean = 10 ± 3) | Percentile | Interpretation |
|---|---|---|---|---|
| Word Discrimination | 27 | 6 | 9 | below average |
| Phonological Segmentation | 22 | 5 | 5 | below average |
| Phonological Blending | 15 | 7 | 16 | average |
| Number Memory Forward | 15 | 8 | 25 | average |
| Number Memory Reversed | 9 | 8 | 25 | average |

| Subtest | Raw Score | Scaled Score (Mean = 10 ± 3) | Percentile | Interpretation |
|---|---|---|---|---|
| Word Memory | 14 | 7 | 16 | average |
| Sentence Memory | 20 | 7 | 16 | average |
| Auditory Comprehension | 21 | 9 | 37 | average |
| Auditory Reasoning | 15 | 10 | 50 | average |

The Word Discrimination subtest assesses the student's ability to discern phonological similarities and differences within word pairs. Phonological Segmentation determines how well a student can manipulate phonemes within words. Those two subtests were the only ones on the TAPS that yielded below-average scores. Phonological Blending determines how well a student can synthesize a word given the individual phonemic sounds. Number Memory Forward (repeating a sequence of numbers) shows how well the student can retain simple sequences of auditory information. Number Memory Reversed and Word Memory show how well the student can retain and manipulate simple sequences of auditory information. Sentence Memory (repeating sentences) shows how well the student can retain details in sentences of increasing length and complexity. Auditory Comprehension (answering questions based on sentences and paragraphs read aloud by the examiner) tests how well the student understands spoken information. Auditory Reasoning is the most complex of the subtests. The auditory cohesion skills for this subtest reflect higher-order linguistic processing, and are related to understanding jokes, riddles, inferences, and abstractions. These items are intended to determine if the student can understand implied meanings, make inferences, or come to logical conclusions given the information in the sentences presented. (Note: subtest descriptions were based on publisher's information.)

The subtest scores may be combined to generate index scores and an overall auditory processing score. Abby's composite scores were:

| Index | Standard Score (Mean = 100 ± 15) | Percentile | Interpretation |
|---|---|---|---|
| Phonologic | 80 | 9 | below average |
| Memory | 88 | 23 | average |
| Cohesion | 98 | 48 | average |
| Overall | 88 | 23 | average |

There was a significant discrepancy between tasks related to phonological skills and others. However, the overall score did not suggest a deficit in auditory processing skills, and Abby did not qualify for language therapy at school because the eligibility is based on the overall score and not on individual subtests or indices. Therefore, even though a deficit in phonological skills was clearly demonstrated, additional testing was necessary.

**The Token Test for Children (TTC).** The TTC is considered a sensitive test of receptive language, memory, and auditory processing skills. On this test, the student follows increasingly complex instructions to manipulate a set of plastic tokens that are five different colors, two sizes, and two shapes. The instructions contain between two and six critical elements that must be held in memory. Instructions for the last subtest also contain sequences of linguistic elements and basic concepts common to classroom and testing instructions.

| Subtest | Raw Score | Scaled Score— Age (Mean = 500 ± 5) | Scaled Score— Grade (Mean = 500 ± 5) | Interpretation |
|---------|-----------|------------------------------------|--------------------------------------|----------------|
| Part I | 9 of 10 | 455 | 474 | below average |
| Part II | 9 of 10 | 496 | 505 | average |
| Part III | 10 of 10 | 502 | 503 | average |
| Part IV | 9 of 10 | 504 | 501 | average |
| Part V | 16 of 21 | 497 | 497 | average |
| Overall | 53 of 61 | 498 | 497 | average |

Abby self-corrected several responses and her performance was average for her age and grade placement. The error on Part I was not significant in terms of skill, although it pulled the subtest score out of the average range. When given the same item a second time, she responded correctly, but the score could not be changed in order to maintain the integrity of the test. Results of this test suggested that receptive language and, specifically, auditory memory were average.

**The Phonological Awareness Test (PAT).** This test was used to gain more detailed information about phonological skills which were identified as a problem area on the TAPS-3, and which directly impact the academic areas of concern: reading and writing. This information should be useful in determining specific goals and objectives for intervention. The problem was that this test is standardized for use with students up to age 9 years, 11 months and she was 5 months older than that. Therefore, Abby was above the chronological age for comparison to a normative group. However, there was not a similar test for her age. Although the norms could not be applied because of her chronological age, the test was used as a criterion-referenced measure. For reference, her performance was compared to the oldest available reference group of 9 years, 11 months old. A child her age would be expected to receive similar or even higher scores than this group. This means that a below-average standard score would likely have been even lower if norms were available for her age. In other words, at worst, this test *overestimated* her skills.

| Subtest | Raw Score | Age Equivalent (CA 10-4) | Percentile (for CA 9-11) | Standard Score* (for CA 9-11) | Interpretation (for CA 9-11) |
|---------|-----------|--------------------------|---------------------------|-------------------------------|------------------------------|
| Rhyming | 19 | 7-0 | 27 | 99 | average |
| Segmentation | 21 | 7-2 | 24 | 90 | average** |
| Isolation | 21 | 6-5 | 11 | 79 | below average |
| Deletion | 14 | 6-8 | 8 | 77 | below average |
| Substitution | 8 | 6-11 | 7 | 72 | below average |
| Blending | 17 | 6-6 | 8 | 75 | below average |
| Graphemes | 40 | 6-11 | 10 | 80 | below average |
| Decoding | 29 | 7-0 | 5 | 67 | below average |
| Total Test | 169 | 6-11 | 5 | 70 | below average |

*Mean = 100 ± 15

**Note that the segmentation score on the PAT was average for a younger child, but a similar task on the TAPS, reported above, indicated that this skill was below average for her age.

This test clearly demonstrated Abby's weakness in manipulating phonological material, both in decoding stimuli presented orally or in writing, and her difficulty in producing phonologically accurate responses. Her overall score on the Phonological Awareness Test was two standard deviations below the mean for a student *below* her chronological age.

Abby had to meet criteria on *two* different language assessments to qualify for language therapy. Her score on the EOWPVT met the criterion. Although the PAT test clearly demonstrated a significant deficiency in phonological awareness, and this was clearly correlated with Abby's difficulty in reading and spelling, she did not qualify for language therapy because she was older than the upper age for this test, the norms could not be applied, and the child study team would not accept the results as representing a low score on a second test of language. Unfortunately, at the time this test was administered, there *was* no comparable test for students her age. Presumably, these deficits should have been diagnosed earlier.

**The Word-R Test.** It was apparent that Abby had a deficit in expressive vocabulary and in phonological skills. However, there were still not two tests of language on which her total score was more than 1.5 standard deviations below the mean. Therefore, this test was administered. It was selected because of the low score on the EWOPVT, to obtain more detailed information about expressive vocabulary skills. The Word-R is a test of expressive vocabulary and semantics and was chosen because the clinician suspected it would yield a low enough score to qualify Abby for language therapy.

| Subtest | Raw Score | Age Equiv. | Percentile | Standard Score | Interpretation |
|---|---|---|---|---|---|
| Associations | 12 | 8–10 | 26 | 92 | average |
| Synonyms | 9 | 8–4 | 7 | 76 | below average |
| Semantic Absurdities | 8 | 7–6 | 7 | 74 | below average |
| Antonyms | 9 | 7–7 | 6 | 72 | below average |
| Definitions | 11 | 7–11 | 17 | 85 | average |
| Multiple Definitions | 9 | 8–6 | 8 | 78 | below average |
| Total Test | 58 | 8–2 | 8 | 73 | below average |

The Associations test required the student to name one of four words that did not go with the others and state why. Synonyms and Antonyms required her to provide a synonym or opposite of the word stated by the examiner. On the Semantic Absurdities subtest, the student hears a sentence and has to correct an error. An example is, "My grandfather is the youngest person in our family." On Definitions, the student provides a definition for a word, and on Multiple Definitions, she gives two different meanings for a word. An example is "bark" (dog sound, part of a tree). Abby's scores on Associations and Definitions were in the average range, but her other scores and the overall test score were below average, indicating a weakness in expressive vocabulary and semantic abilities.

## Summary

Abby was a 10-year, 4-month old girl in fourth grade. She received speech therapy and mastered production of /s/. Her teachers and parents stated that reading and writing skills improved, but she continued to have significant difficulty with reading decoding and writing. Therefore, she was seen for a complete speech and language evaluation. Her speech was characterized by persistent errors on production of /r/ and /r/ blends, coproduction of /f/ and /th/ for /th/ at the end of words, and interdental tongue placement for /t, d, n, l/. Results of two tests (and several subtests of other tests) of expressive vocabulary, semantic abilities, and phonological skills were below the 10th percentile. Receptive vocabulary, auditory memory, and other auditory processing skills were average. Resonance was moderately hypernasal.

## Recommendation

Because of her scores below the 10th percentile on tests of articulation, expressive vocabulary, and semantic skills, Abby was eligible for speech and language services. It was recommended that Abby receive articulation and language therapy three times per week, in a small group no larger than two students, for 30 minutes, in order to improve expressive vocabulary, semantic skills, phonological skills, and articulation as described above. A home program to reinforce skills on a daily basis was also recommended. She was also underwent pharyngeal flap surgery and post-operative resonance was normal.

## SUMMARY

In summary, children with VCFS are likely to have speech and language disorders, and the pattern of these disorders may be syndrome-specific. Most of these children receive speech and language therapy in school, and the school-based speech specialist must be prepared to provide a thorough evaluation, develop a detailed IEP, implement treatment at school, and develop a home program for practice and reinforcement. Therapy must be frequent, children should be seen on an individual basis or seen groups no larger than two, and therapy procedures must be direct and organized. With these provisions, therapy can be successful in establishing normal articulation skills. Language skills, especially in the area of pragmatic and social communication, may require ongoing training and support throughout school to be sure the student's language skills mature with the increasing linguistic demands that are a natural part of maturation.

## REFERENCES

Boone, D. R., McFarlane, S. C., & Von Berg, S. L. (2004). *The voice and voice therapy* (7th ed.). Boston: Allyn and Bacon.

Chegar, B. E., Tatum, S. A., III, Marrinan, E., & Shprintzen, R. J. (2006). Upper airway asymmetry in velo-cardio-facial syndrome. *International Journal of Pediatric Otorhinolaryngology*, 70(8), 1375–1381.

Christensen, M., & Hanson, M. (1981). An investigation of the efficacy of oral myofunctional therapy for pre-first grade children. *Journal of Speech and Hearing Disorders*, 46(2), 160–165.

Golding, K. J. (1980, March). The relationship between speech therapy and surgery in the treatment of "cleft palate" speech. Annual symposium of the Center for Craniofacial Disorders of Montefiore Hospital and Medical Center and the Albert Einstein College of Medicine, Bronx, NY.

Golding-Kushner, K. J. (1991). *Craniofacial morphology and velopharyngeal function in four syndromes of clefting*. Unpublished doctoral dissertation, the Graduate School and University Center, City University of New York, New York.

Golding-Kushner, K. J. (1995). Treatment of articulation and resonance disorders associated with cleft palate and VPI. In R. J. Shprintzen & J. Bardach (Eds.), *Cleft palate speech management: A multidisciplinary approach* (pp. 327–351), St. Louis, MO: C. V. Mosby.

Golding-Kushner, K. J. (2001). *Therapy techniques for cleft palate speech and VPI*. San Diego, CA: Singular Publishing Group.

Golding-Kushner, K. (2005). Speech and language disorders in velo-cardio-facial syndrome. In K. Murphy & P. Scambler (Eds.), *Velo-cardio-facial syndrome: A model for understanding microdeletion disorders* (pp. 181–199), Cambridge, UK: Cambridge University Press.

Hodson, B., & Paden, E. (1991). *Targeting intelligible speech* (2nd ed.). Austin, TX: Pro-Ed.

Landsman, D. (2004). *Impact of VCFS on learning and school performance*. 10th annual international meeting of the Velo-Cardio-Facial Syndrome Educational Foundation, Inc., and the Fourth International Conference for 22q11.2 Deletions, Atlanta, GA.

Landsman. D, (2006, July). *Educational interventions for children with VCFS*. 12th Annual International Scientific Meeting of the Velo-Cardio-Facial Syndrome Educational Foundation, Inc., Strasbourg, France.

Peterson-Falzon, S. J., Hardin-Jones, M. A., & Karnell, M. J. (2001). *Cleft palate speech* (3rd ed.). St. Louis, MO: Mosby.

Peterson-Falzone, S. J., Trost-Cardamone, J. E., Karnell, M. P., & Hardin-Jones, M. A. (2006). *The clinician's guide for treating cleft palate speech*. St. Louis, MO: Mosby.

Powers, G., & Starr, C. D. (1974). The effects of muscle exercises on velopharyngeal gap and nasality. *Cleft Palate Journal, 11*, 28–35.

Rubin, J. S., Sataloff, R. T., & Korovin, G. S. (2006). *Diagnosis and treatment of voice disorders* (3rd ed.). San Diego, CA: Plural Publishing.

Ruscello, D. M. (1982). A selected review of palatal training procedures. *Cleft Palate Journal, 18*, 181–193.

Shprintzen, R. J. (2005). Velo-cardio-facial syndrome. In S. B. Cassidy & J. E. Allanson (Eds.), *Management of genetic syndromes* (pp. 615–632), Hoboken, NJ: Wiley-Liss.

Starr, C. D. (1990). Treatment by therapeutic exercises. In J. Bardach & H. L. Morris (Eds.), *Multidisciplinary management of cleft lip and palate* (pp. 792–798). Philadelphia: W. B. Saunders.

Traquina, D., Golding-Kushner, K. J., & Shprintzen, R. J. (December 1990). Comparison of tonsil size based on oral and nasopharyngoscopic observation. Society of Ear Nose and Throat Advances in Children, Washington, DC.

Van Demark, D. R., and Hardin, M. A. (1990). Speech therapy for the child with cleft lip and palate. In J. Bardach & H. L. Morris (Eds.), *Multidisciplinary management of cleft lip and palate* (pp. 799–806). Philadelphia: W. B. Saunders.

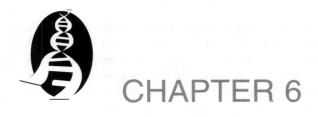

# CHAPTER 6

# Childhood Illness in VCFS and Its Impact on School Attendance and Performance

## ANNE MARIE HIGGINS, RN, FNP, MA

$M$ost school-aged children with VCFS experience many more infections and illnesses than children in the general population. These illnesses can be caused by anatomical abnormalities in the body as well as immune and endocrine system dysfunction. The anatomical abnormalities include a small or absent thymus; craniofacial structural abnormalities of the ears and throat; lung and heart abnormalities; and gastrointestinal, muscular, and skeletal abnormalities. This chapter will discuss how complex health problems associated with VCFS can have a negative impact on school attendance and performance.

To keep the body healthy and disease free, a functioning immune system is essential. The immune system is made up of organs (e.g., thymus, tonsils, adenoids), tissues (e.g., bone marrow, lymphatic tissue, skin), and cells (e.g., plasma, white blood cells, red blood cells). These components work together to defend the body from invading organisms or foreign substances. The immune system must recognize what is an invading organism such as a virus or bacteria or a harmless foreign substance such as pollen. The immune system also has to differentiate between what is self and what is not self. When the immune system is unable to differentiate self from non-self, an autoimmune disorder can develop. The four major functioning parts of the immune system are made up of specialized cells called phagocytes, complement, B-lymphocytes, and T-lymphocytes. The B-lymphocytes make up what is called the humoral immune system and the T-lymphocytes make up the cellular immune system. These parts function differently within a complex system of overlaps and back-ups. The phagocyte function and complement are part of the innate or inborn, nonspecific immunity and are usually normal in VCFS. The B-lymphocytes and T-lymphocytes are part of the acquired or specific immunity. The B-lymphocytes mature in the bone marrow and produce antibodies or immunoglobulins. Antibodies are proteins that the body makes in response to an invading organism such as a bacteria or virus. Antibodies are also produced in response to an immunization. The T-lymphocytes mature in the thymus and are essential for orchestrating much of the immune response by telling other cells what to do. In VCFS, if an immune dysfunction is found, it is usually a problem with the function of the humoral or cellular system.

Normal immune system function changes over a lifetime. The early immune system function depends upon innate immunity and is also dependent upon specific antibodies acquired in the womb by the infant from the mother. The mother passes her acquired antibodies through the placenta to help protect the infant from illness. The mother's antibodies decrease in the infant over several months of life and the infant must make its own antibodies as it is exposed to organisms or vaccines. The thymus is an organ in the chest that is responsible for a portion of the immune system function in infancy and early childhood. Some infants with VCFS are born without a thymus or the thymus can be totally or partially removed during heart surgery leading to poor immune system function. In some instances, residual thymic tissue can be present elsewhere in the body and the immune system function remains intact. A functioning thymus or thymic tissue is needed so the child can develop protection against certain illnesses and respond to some childhood vaccines. As a child grows older, the thymus is not as important in fighting infection as other parts of the immune system (i.e., bone marrow, lymph system). A functioning immune system and proper response to childhood vaccines are important for achieving resistance to disease as well as reducing susceptibility to childhood illness. In general, immune system abnormalities are common in VCFS but the most severe immune deficiencies are uncommon. It is also uncommon to have severe or life-threatening infections; however, almost every child with VCFS has a mild or moderate problem with the way the immune system functions. A child with VCFS with mild immune system abnormalities usually has a history of frequent upper respiratory infections and is not at risk for more severe infections. A child with VCFS and moderate immune abnormalities usually has more frequent lower respiratory infections and is at risk for developing chronic lung disease. If a child with VCFS has not had many infections in infancy and childhood, the likelihood for an immune abnormality later in life is rare.

In VCFS, an immune evaluation including a physical examination by an immunologist and specialized laboratory testing is important in the first year of life, especially prior to receiving any live virus vaccines. The specific laboratory testing depends upon the child's age and immunization history. A younger infant's immune evaluation includes a complete blood count with differential and platelets and an assessment of the total numbers of antibodies or immunoglobulins in the blood as well as total numbers of T-lymphocytes, also known as lymphocyte subsets. In VCFS, if an immune disorder is found, it is usually seen as low numbers of the T-lymphocyte subsets called CD4 and CD8 cells. CD4 cells are the "helper cells" that help orchestrate the other immune cells to function. CD8 cells are important for fighting viral and bacterial infections. Low numbers of these T-cells can lead to "opportunistic infections" that usually do not cause disease in a person with a normal immune system. Treatment includes prophylactic antibiotics to prevent these possible life-threatening infections. Often these antibiotics can be stopped when immune system function improves as the child gets older.

The specific laboratory testing to determine if the recommended 12- to 15-month live virus vaccines can be given includes a complete blood count with differential and platelets and a measure of the total numbers of immuno-globulins and acquired antibodies to vaccines received as well as an assessment of the number and function of lymphocytes in the blood. If the number of lymphocytes is low but the function is normal, it is usually fine to give live virus vaccines. If the number of lymphocytes is normal but the function is abnormal, live virus vaccines should not be given. The key element is the function of the cells rather than the number. With a lymphocyte functional abnormality, a child with VCFS may have a poor response to vaccines or may have an adverse reaction. A reaction could be localized skin rash, fever, general body rash, or an infection with the live virus in the vaccine. If a child with VCFS is over 1 year of age when seen by an immunologist, is up to date on all immunizations including live virus vaccines, and has not had any adverse reactions, then laboratory testing and interventions should be based upon the child's history of infections. If there is no history of recurrent infections, a measurable immune disorder may not be found. Although rare, if an immune disorder is discovered and persists, monthly intravenous antibodies to boost the immune system may be needed. In VCFS, immune system dysfunction usually improves with age. It is possible, however, that persistent immune dys-function can contribute to the development of recurrent or chronic infections throughout the school years. While a formal immune system evaluation before school age is optimum, it is important to note that laboratory testing can be normal and a child with VCFS may still have problems with recurrent infections.

Recurrent upper respiratory infections (URIs) are the most common and account for most outpatient visits and school absences in children. School-aged children in the general population have 2 to 7 upper respiratory infections during a typical school year, whereas children with VCFS can have more than

10. Frequent ear and sinus infections, colds, sore throats, and flulike illnesses are common in VCFS. Frequent ear infections and ear fluid can be attributed to immune system dysfunction coupled with the craniofacial abnormality of narrow ear canals typical in VCFS. Children with VCFS often require the surgical intervention of pressure equalization ear tubes. Even though many children with VCFS have more frequent ear infections than normal children, antibiotics are not always helpful and can lead to antibiotic resistance. Treatment guidelines by the American Academy of Pediatrics based upon symptoms and the child's age should be followed (http://www.aap.org/healthtopics/ear infections.cfm). Hearing loss is also common in VCFS due to congenital neurological abnormalities and/or frequent infections and fluid. It is important for every child with VCFS to have an initial hearing evaluation in infancy or early childhood at the latest. If hearing loss is found, frequent assessments, proper treatment, and follow-up are needed. Normal hearing is essential to speech, social development, and school performance.

Tonsils and adenoids are part of the lymphatic immune system that can become inflamed and enlarged in response to frequent URIs. This inflammatory immune response may cause increased susceptibility to infection and problems with sleep due to airway obstruction. These problems can occur in the general population; however, they are usually more severe in VCFS. Hypotonia or low muscle tone in VCFS is a structural abnormality that contributes to problems throughout the body. The tonsils are attached to the muscles in the throat and are usually seen when a child says "Ahhhh." Because of low muscle tone in VCFS, the tonsils can extend abnormally down into the throat where they cannot be fully visualized on oral exam. To assess the true size and position of the tonsils, a fiberoptic endoscopy is required. Enlarged and/or abnormally placed tonsils can cause airway obstruction even without infection. A tonsillectomy can usually alleviate these airway problems and sleep disturbance. Adenoids can be useful for speech production in VCFS and should not be removed without appropriate consultation by a health care practitioner knowledgeable about VCFS.

The majority of URIs are caused by viruses, yet there is a common misconception that colored nasal secretions mean bacterial infection. The color of the secretions is actually caused by a chemical reaction in the body to any invading pathogen, virus or bacteria. White blood cells cluster to defend the body from the pathogen and the chemical reaction produces a substance similar to chlorine. Chlorine is what colors a swimming pool green, hence, the green color of secretions. This color misconception leads to the all too common practice of using antibiotics to treat viral illness. The unnecessary use of antibiotics can in turn lead to further illness by destroying healthy bacteria and promoting antibiotic resistance. It is important for parents and health care professionals to understand that appropriate treatment for most URIs does not include antibiotics. There are many over-the-counter medicines to treat viral URIs or simply good old-fashioned home remedies, TLC, and tincture of time. The best indicator for proper diagnosis of a bacterial infection is duration and severity of symptoms. A viral URI can last up to two weeks with varying symptoms of sneezing, coughing, runny nose, and mild fever; however, a child is often able to function in school. If a viral illness is prolonged and there is no improvement in symptoms over time, children can develop secondary bacterial infections. When a bacterial illness is diagnosed, it is important to treat with the appropriate antibiotic, a common narrow-spectrum medication versus one of the newer "designer drugs." Parents of children with VCFS express frustration with frequent pediatrician visits and the perceived need for multiple antibiotics when their children do not recover after one treatment course. It is important to note that a child with VCFS can have multiple URIs in a row. Each illness puts the child at risk for subsequent infection by taxing the immune system and irritating the lining of the nose and throat. As a result, parents often ask for a "stronger" antibiotic with each new illness, thus increasing the risk for antibiotic resistance even further. This cycle of frequent illness and the use of inappropriate treatments can leave a child vulnerable should a more serious infection occur. Antibiotic resistance means that the bacteria or other invading pathogen that caused an illness changes so that the antibiotic is no longer effective. The Centers for Disease Control and Prevention has an ongoing campaign that provides important information about antibiotic resistance and the proper use of antibiotics (http://www.cdc.gov/drugresistance/). Because children with VCFS often have complex medical problems, it is important for parents and health care practitioners to work together to determine the need for the proper medical interventions.

Lower respiratory tract infections (LRIs) such as pneumonia, bronchitis, and bronchiolitis (croup) are more common in infancy and early childhood. When a child with VCFS has a history of frequent LRIs and multiple hospitalizations in the first year of life, the degree of immune system dysfunction is more significant and there is the potential for repeat hospitalizations. If a child with VCFS is not admitted to the hospital with these types of infections during the first year of life, then the risk of hospitalization in subsequent years is generally decreased. Medical interventions for an immune deficiency are varied and depend upon the degree of immune dysfunction. Prophylactic antibiotics to prevent pneumonia and repeat doses of vaccines are the most common interventions, whereas intravenous antibodies to boost the immune system are less common. Usually these interventions are limited to early childhood but can extend into the school years. If lower respiratory illnesses continue in older children with VCFS, long absences from school including hospitalization may be required. It is important to note that prophylactic antibiotics in later childhood are generally not useful for preventing LRIs and URIs and in fact can contribute to a decrease in immune function and an increase in antibiotic resistance. Inappropriate use of antibiotics can decrease the normal protections in the respiratory and gastrointestinal tracts by killing useful bacteria and allowing the growth of antibiotic-resistant bacteria.

Children with VCFS can also develop fevers of unknown origin or unusually low body temperatures that are puzzling for health care practitioners, parents, and school personnel. This inability to regulate body temperature in VCFS is thought to be due to an imbalance in the central nervous system; however, these children are often unnecessarily treated for infection. Children with VCFS can also have allergies and asthma causing chronic upper and lower respiratory tract symptoms that occur over many years even with proper treatments. Less common, urinary tract infections can occur due to structural abnormalities in the kidney. If a child with VCFS isn't considered ill enough to stay home, frequent school nurse visits for medications and/or treatments can interrupt classroom time.

Often a child with VCFS is also diagnosed with DiGeorge syndrome; these two are used interchangeably but they are not the same. A person can have VCFS and not DiGeorge and vice versa. DiGeorge is not a syndrome but a sequence or triad of symptoms that include congenital heart abnormality, absent or partial thymus causing immune dysfunction, and parathyroid disorder causing hypocalcemia and possible seizures (http://www.vcfsef.org/articles/en/pdf/NAMEGAME.PDF).

It is possible to have VCFS and only one or two of these three symptoms; this is often referred to as partial DiGeorge. Generally, immune dysfunction and hypocalcemia lessen with age but can present variably throughout life. Congenital heart abnormalities in VCFS often require surgical correction. While surgery can lead to complete resolution of the abnormality, sometimes there are residual problems in cardiac function throughout life.

Because VCFS can affect every body system, many children undergo multiple operations to correct various anatomical abnormalities. Surgical repair of the heart and vascular system, craniofacial structures (ears, palate, and throat), and gastrointestinal tract are the most common in infancy and childhood. While it is optimum to have these operations prior to the start of school, it may not always be possible. Abnormalities of the spine (e.g., scoliosis) may be seen in early school years and progress as the child gets older. Surgical intervention, if needed, is usually postponed until the post-pubertal growth spurt in adolescence. Some abnormalities in VCFS require multiple operations that extend through the school years and occasionally into adulthood. Surgery, hospitalization, and the recovery period clearly have an adverse effect on school attendance. Every surgical procedure and anesthesia carry the potential for complications and a possible setback in the normal quality of life. It is important to note that there can be postoperative residual problems with heart and circulatory function that can affect strength and stamina throughout life. The optimum goal of corrective surgery for speech disorders is normal speech and minimal or no upper airway obstruction. When there is airway obstruction, sleep can be disturbed which in turn can affect vitality and school performance. Airway obstruction can also cause diminished strength and stamina during physical activity requiring exertion, such as physical education class or sports. At the most severe end, children with VCFS who experience airway obstruction cannot climb stairs or participate in normal playtime activities. Even with successful surgery to correct speech and hearing, most children with VCFS carry individualized educational plans (IEP) that require time out of the regular classroom for special education interventions.

Some children with VCFS develop autoimmune diseases related to immune system dysfunction such as juvenile rheumatoid arthritis (JRA), skin disorders (i.e., psoriasis), and thyroid disorders (i.e., hypothyroidism and Graves' disease—autoimmune hyperthyroidism). While it has not been studied extensively in VCFS, the likelihood of an autoimmune disease may be higher if an immune disorder was found in early childhood. Autoimmune disorders commonly occur in later childhood to early adolescence. Each of these autoimmune disorders has the potential for causing discomfort and disability that can affect participation in school and extracurricular activities. JRA symptoms of joint pain and immobility can be variable with episodic flareups over time. Skin disorders not only cause discomfort but embarrassment at a time when peer acceptance is crucial. Excessive tiredness or irritability and hyperactivity can clearly affect the ability to focus and learn. All of these symptoms can be present in VCFS but be caused by neuropsychological disorders such as ADHD or OCD rather than a thyroid disorder. Proper diagnosis and treatment of all autoimmune disorders is therefore essential.

The endocrine system regulates hormones and metabolic processes in the body. Children with VCFS can have problems regulating calcium and glucose resulting in seizures on the most severe end to nausea, tiredness, and general malaise on the less severe end. Headaches and gastrointestinal complaints are common in all school-aged children but can be more severe in VCFS. While there can be a psychosomatic component to many of these complaints, it is important to explore all possible physiological causes in children with VCFS. Headaches can be due to jaw abnormalities such as temporomandibular joint malformation or vascular malformations leading to migraines. Thrombocytopenia, a bleeding disorder, has been found to be more common after puberty. Psychological and psychiatric symptoms also increase after puberty in VCFS. It is unclear how hormonal changes affect the body systems in VCFS but it is important for parents, school personnel, and health care practitioners to monitor new symptoms as children reach adolescence.

Almost all children with VCFS are born with some degree of hypotonia (low muscle tone). The degree of hypotonia, whether it is mild, moderate, or severe, determines the impact on a child's life. Fine and gross motor milestones are generally delayed in VCFS due in part to low muscle tone. Children with VCFS may have difficulties with grasping, drawing, and legible writing. Hand coordination, writing, and drawing usually improve over time. Parents often describe clumsiness in walking and running. While muscle tone usually improves with age, school-aged children with VCFS can have problems with balance and stamina especially during physical education and sports participation. Structural abnormalities of the feet, legs, and hands can also affect school and sports participation. Children with VCFS often complain of leg pains and cramping with or without weight bearing activity. Parents can assist with simple stretching and massage for leg and foot pain associated with hypotonia. Properly fitting, supportive shoes with soft insoles are better tolerated than hard orthotics. Some orthopedic interventions and occasionally surgical interventions can assist with foot abnormalities. Many children with VCFS receive physical and occupational therapies that take them out of the classroom. These modalities offer varying degrees of improvement because the hypotonia and structural abnormalities are congenital and can be lifelong regardless of intervention. If a child with VCFS cannot participate and keep up with peers in a team sport, activities such as horseback riding or karate can be a better choice and measure for individual success.

It is well documented that there are varying degrees of learning disabilities associated with VCFS. Frequent school absences due to illness, surgery, and the need for interventions outside the classroom can negatively impact the educational experience of children with VCFS. Educators, parents, and health care professionals must be cognizant of the multiple factors involved in the potential for these children's success in school and in life.

The Velo-Cardio-Facial Syndrome Specialist Fact Sheet below lists all anomalies that have been seen in VCFS (http://www.vcfsef.org/articles/en/pdf/factsheet.PDF). No person has all of these anomalies and each anomaly can have a variable presentation in each individual. This variable presentation can have different effects on each individual's abilities as well as limitations. Some anomalies are present at birth; others emerge over the lifespan. Most people with VCFS have between 10 and 20 anomalies. The most common anomalies include cardiac defects, hypocalcemia, craniofacial anomalies, feeding problems, constipation, palate anomalies, speech disorders, immune dysfunction, hypotonia, fine and gross motor developmental delays, learning disabilities, and behavioral and psychological concerns. It is important that treatments and interventions be carefully planned with parents, educators, and health care practitioners to meet an individual's specific needs throughout life. While limitations can be difficult, the plan for future success in life and livelihood for someone with VCFS should take into consideration the most important factor for continued success . . . satisfaction with one's unique abilities.

## VELO-CARDIO-FACIAL SYNDROME SPECIALIST FACT SHEET

*Velo-cardio-facial syndrome* (VCFS) is caused by a deletion of a small segment of the long arm of chromosome 22. It is one of the most common genetic disorders in humans. The following list shows the anomalies that have been found in VCFS. No features are found in 100% of cases, but all occur with sufficient frequency to warrant assessment. If you have any questions, or if you would like to learn more about VCFS, you may reach the Velo-Cardio-Facial Syndrome Educational Foundation, Inc. by telephone at 315-464-6590, by fax at 315-464-5321, or by email at vcfsef@mail.upstate.edu. The foundation maintains a Web site at www.vcfsef.org.

## Craniofacial/Oral Findings

1. Overt, submucous, or occult submucous cleft palate
2. Retrognathia (retruded lower jaw)
3. Platybasia (flat skull base)
4. Asymmetric crying facies in infancy
5. Structurally asymmetric face
6. Functionally asymmetric face
7. Vertical maxillary excess (long face)
8. Straight facial profile
9. Congenitally missing teeth (one or several)
10. Small teeth
11. Enamel hypoplasia (primary dentition)
12. Hypotonic, flaccid facies
13. Downturned oral commissures
14. Cleft lip (uncommon)
15. Microcephaly
16. Small posterior cranial fossa

## Eye Findings

17. Tortuous retinal vessels
18. Suborbital congestion ("allergic shiners")
19. Strabismus
20. Narrow palpebral fissures
21. Posterior embryotoxon
22. Small optic disk
23. Prominent corneal nerves
24. Cataract
25. Iris nodules
26. Iris coloboma (uncommon)
27. Retinal coloboma (uncommon)

28. Small eyes

29. Mild orbital hypertelorism

30. Mild vertical orbital dystopia

31. Puffy upper eyelids

## Ear/Hearing Findings

32. Overfolded helix

33. Attached lobules

34. Protuberant, cup-shaped ears

35. Small ears

36. Mildly asymmetric ears

37. Frequent otitis media

38. Mild conductive hearing loss

39. Sensorineural hearing loss (often unilateral)

40. Ear tags or pits (uncommon)

41. Narrow external ear canals

## Nasal Findings

42. Prominent nasal bridge

43. Bulbous nasal tip

44. Mildly separated nasal domes (nasal tip appears bifid)

45. Pinched alar base, narrow nostrils

46. Narrow nasal passages

## Cardiac and Thoracic Vascular Findings

47. VSD (ventricular septal defect)

48. ASD (atrial septal defect)

49. Pulmonic atresia or stenosis

50. Tetralogy of Fallot

51. Right-sided aorta

52. Truncus arteriosus

53. PDA (patent ductus arteriosus)

54. Interrupted aorta, type B

55. Coarctation of the aorta

56. Aortic valve anomalies

57. Aberrant subclavian arteries

58. Vascular ring

59. Anomalous origin of carotid artery

60. Transposition of the great vessels

61. Tricuspid atresia

## Vascular Anomalies

62. Medially displaced internal carotid arteries

63. Tortuous or kinked internal carotids

64. Jugular vein anomalies

65. Absence of internal carotid artery (unilateral)

66. Absence of vertebral artery (unilateral)

67. Low bifurcation of common carotid

68. Tortuous or kinked vertebral arteries

69. Raynaud's phenomenon

70. Small veins

71. Circle of Willis anomalies

## Neurologic, Brain, and MR Findings

72. Periventricular cysts (mostly at anterior horns)

73. Small cerebellar vermis

74. Cerebellar hypoplasia/dysgenesis

75. White matter UBOs (unidentified bright objects)

76. Generalized hypotonia

77. Cerebellar ataxia

78. Seizures

79. Strokes

80. Spina bifida/meningomyelocele

81. Mild developmental delay

82. Enlarged Sylvian fissure

### Pharyngeal/Laryngeal/Airway Findings

83. Upper airway obstruction in infancy

84. Absent or small adenoids

85. Laryngeal web (anterior)

86. Large pharyngeal airway

87. Laryngomalacia

88. Arytenoid hyperplasia

89. Pharyngeal hypotonia

90. Asymmetric pharyngeal movement

91. Thin pharyngeal muscle

92. Unilateral vocal cord paresis

93. Reactive airway disease

94. Asthma

### Abdominal/Kidney/Gut

95. Hypoplastic/aplastic kidney

96. Cystic kidneys

97. Inguinal hernias

98. Umbilical hernias

99. Malrotation of bowel

100. Diastasis recti

101. Diaphragmatic hernia (uncommon)

102. Hirschsprung megacolon (rare)

## Limb Findings

103. Small hands and feet

104. Tapered digits

105. Short nails

106. Rough, red, scaly skin on hands and feet

107. Morphea

108. Contractures

109. Triphalangeal thumbs

110. Polydactyly, both pre- and postaxial (uncommon)

111. Soft tissue syndactyly

## Problems in Infancy

112. Feeding difficulty, failure to thrive

113. Nasal vomiting

114. Gastroesophageal reflux

115. Irritability

116. Chronic constipation (not Hirschsprung megacolon)

## Genitourinary

117. Hypospadias

118. Cryptorchidism

119. Vesico-ureteral reflux

## Speech/Language

120. Severe hypernasality

121. Severe articulation impairment (glottal stops)

122. Language impairment (usually mild delay)

123. Velopharyngeal insufficiency (usually severe)

124. High-pitched voice

125. Hoarseness

## Cognitive/Learning

126. Learning disabilities (math concept, reading comprehension)

127. Concrete thinking, difficulty with abstraction

128. Drop in IQ scores in school years (test artifact)

129. Borderline normal intellect

130. Occasional mild mental retardation

131. Attention deficit hyperactivity disorder

## Miscellaneous Anomalies

132. Spontaneous oxygen desaturation without apnea

133. Thrombocytopenia, Bernard-Soulier disease

134. Juvenile rheumatoid arthritis

135. Poor body temperature regulation

## Psychiatric/Psychological

136. Bipolar affective disorder

137. Manic depressive illness and psychosis

138. Rapid or ultrarapid cycling of mood disorder

139. Mood disorder

140. Depression

141. Hypomania

142. Schizoaffective disorder

143. Schizophrenia

144. Impulsiveness

145. Flat affect

146. Dysthymia

147. Cyclothymia

148. Social immaturity

149. Obsessive-compulsive disorder

150. Generalized anxiety disorder

151. Phobias

152. Severe startle response

## Immunologic

153. Frequent upper respiratory infections

154. Frequent lower airway disease (pneumonia, bronchitis)

155. Reduced T-cell populations

156. Reduced thymic hormone

## Endocrine

157. Hypocalcemia

158. Hypoparathyroidism

159. Hypothyroidism

160. Mild growth deficiency, relatively small stature

161. Absent, hypoplastic thymus

162. Small pituitary gland (rare)

## Skeletal/Muscle/Orthopedic

163. Scoliosis

164. Spina bifida occulta

165. Hemivertebrae

166. Butterfly vertebrae

167. Fused vertebrae (usually cervical)

168. Osteopenia

169. Sprengel's anomaly, scapular deformation

170. Talipes equinovarus

171. Small skeletal muscles

172. Joint dislocations

173. Chronic leg pains

174. Flat foot arches

175. Hyperextensible/lax joints

176. Rib fusion

177. Extra ribs

178. Tethered cord

179. Syrinx

### Skin/Integument

180. Abundant scalp hair

181. Thin-appearing skin (venous patterns easily visible)

### Secondary Sequences/Associations

182. Robin sequence

183. DiGeorge sequence

184. Potter sequence

185. CHARGE association

186. Holoprosencephaly (single case)

### Some Other Facts about the Syndrome:

Population prevalence (estimated): 1:2,000 people

Birth incidence (estimated): 1:1,800 births

Prevalence in infants with conotruncal heart anomalies: 30%

Prevalence in cleft palate (without cleft lip): 8%

## BIBLIOGRAPHY/SUGGESTED READINGS

Cunningham, C. *Immunology.* Presentation at the 10th annual meeting of the Velo-Cardio-Facial Syndrome Education Association; New York. Available from: http://www.conferencemediagroup.com/detail.asp?product_id=VC-04-01-13

Domachowske, J. *Pediatric issues.* Presentation at the 11th annual meeting of the Velo-Cardio-Facial Syndrome Education Association; New York. Available from: http://www.conferencemediagroup.com/detail.asp?product_id=VC-05-01-03 http://www.vcfsef.org

Sullivan, K. (2005). Immunodeficiency in velo-cardio-facial syndrome. In K. Murphy & P. Scambler (Eds.), *Velo-cardio-facial syndrome: A model for understanding micro-deletion disorders* (pp. 123–134). Cambridge/New York: Cambridge University Press.

VCFS Educational Foundation International Scientific Meeting. Conference audiotapes. (audiotapes can be ordered through http://www.conferencemediagroup.com/)

# PART II

# Educational Interventions and Evaluation of Effective Practices

## DONNA CUTLER-LANDSMAN, MS

*T*he second part of this book focuses on educational interventions. There are virtually no formal scientific studies that have been done looking at the effectiveness of educational interventions and the VCFS population. This poses an ethical dilemma. Should recommendations be made when no formal studies have been conducted to support the suggestions? Some members of the scientific research community may not think so, but parents and teachers needing assistance today are not willing to wait many years until the formal studies are conducted and evaluated and new theories emerge. The children with VCFS in school, today, deserve more.

In order to compile this book, great care was used to research suggested programs and interventions. The Council of Exceptional Children, the What Works Clearinghouse (a Department of Education initiative to evaluate teaching practices), the National Panel of Teachers of Reading report, and the National Council of Teachers of Mathematics are just some of the sources consulted. In addition, parents and teachers of students with VCFS provided valuable information as to their experiences with programs and interventions as did educators with many years of teaching experience.

## EVALUATION OF EDUCATIONAL INTERVENTIONS

It is vitally important that anyone using this book to design a program for a child with VCFS use ongoing assessment methods to determine if the educational interventions chosen are working. There is a wide range of variability between students with VCFS and no one particular program will be best for everyone. The Council of Exceptional Children Alert series suggests the use of formative evaluation to measure the effectiveness of specific interventions (Espin, Shin, & Busch, 2000). Formative evaluation uses ongoing collection of information to evaluate instructional implementations and then make modifications to better meet students' needs.

There are two approaches to formative evaluation and each provides different types of data (Fuchs & Deno, 1991). The first measures specific sub-skill mastery or short-term learning goals, and the second focuses on global outcomes or desired terminal behavior. The two approaches answer different questions. The short-term measurement answers the question, "Has the student learned the skill just recently taught?" For example, is the student able to blend sounds? The general outcome measurement answers the question, "Has learning this skill led to growth and improvement in the academic area involved?" In this sense, has learning to blend sounds resulted in an overall improvement in reading ability?

There are four prominent approaches to formative evaluation:

- Curriculum-based assessment (CBA)—This approach involves observing and recording progress in a school curriculum using pre- and post-testing in a published curriculum or with teacher-made tests. As students master subsets of skills they then move on to more advanced skills in the hierarchy. This is an example of the sub-skill or short-term approach to formative evaluation.

- Curriculum-based measurement (CBM)—This is a progress monitoring system in which student performance is measured at least weekly with materials that represent an entire curricular domain (such as reading). This approach is a clear example of the general outcome approach to formative evaluation. Student progress is measured with reliable instruments throughout an instructional program and adjustments are made if progress is insufficient.

- Portfolio assessment—This is the collection of student work that represents what the student has done in the classroom and infers what the students can do. It relies on teacher identified "authentic" tasks that simulate what the student will need to succeed in the "real" world. In portfolio assessment the student performance is judged on the basis of the tasks the teacher deems important learning outcomes.

■ Performance assessment—In performance assessment, student competence is measured in real or simulated situations rather than with paper/pencil tasks. The teacher determines the frequency and the manner in which these assessments indicate a need for adjustments to the educational program.

Research on formative evaluation suggests that two additional components contribute to an educational program's effectiveness (L. S. Fuchs & D. Fuchs, 1986). First, it is important to collect data and analyze it at frequent intervals. It is also important to have specified rules to interpret this data, rather than to rely on teacher judgment alone. An example of a specified rule might be: If a student's score is below the 70th percentile on a measure for three consecutive days, change the method of instructional delivery. The second component that contributes to promoting student achievement is graphing the data as opposed to simply recording it. Graphs help educators view progress pictorially and assist in identifying trends. They can also provide motivating feedback to the student.

Of the four methods discussed earlier, both curriculum-based assessment (CBA) and curriculum-based measurement (CBM) use data collection and graphing measurement. In terms of reliability and validity of the measures, CBM has the strongest empirical database and has been researched extensively at the elementary level (Espin et al., 2000). This method, however, does not provide information as to how to change instruction when students are not progressing. The other methods, CBA, portfolio and performance assessments, do more readily provide feedback on methods, but using measures developed by individual teachers is less reliable.

In terms of the VCFS student, it is essential that teachers use careful and frequent data collection to determine the effectiveness of their teaching methods. Parents should insist that the schools show evidence of progress with the instructional program chosen. A combination of CBM measurements and CBA, portfolio, and performance instruments might provide the richest data source by which to base curricular decisions. In addition, it would be best if teachers do assessments at least biweekly, so that several weeks or months don't pass before a change in instructional methods can be instituted. This is particularly important considering the difficulty many schools experience programming successfully for the child with VCFS.

It is also important for parents and schools to work closely together to determine the effectiveness of the interventions in view of the overall child. Children with VCFS have multiple issues to address, and there will need to be a balance between allowing the child to play and relax at home versus the need to remediate skills or attend therapy sessions. Many parents of children with VCFS complain of hours of homework a night, frustrating study sessions, and failing grades at school. Keeping up with the demands of the school day is extremely challenging for these children, so all parties involved will need to frequently assess the suitability of the programs chosen.

I have included a general bibliography at the end of this section of books that pertain to educating special needs children and that have relevance for the VCFS population and offer additional suggestions for interventions. At the end of each age level are additional book suggestions that are particularly applicable for that stage in the child's development.

## REFERENCES

Espin, C., Shin, J., & Busch, T. (2000). Focusing on formative evaluation, *Current Practice Alerts: The Division of Learning Disabilities and Division for Research of the Council of Exceptional Children*, Issue 3.

Fuchs, L. S., & Deno, L. S. (1991). Paradigmatic distinction between instructionally relevant measurement models. *Exceptional Children, 57,* 488–500.

Fuchs, L. S., & Fuchs, D. (1986). Effects of systematic formative evaluation: A Meta-analysis, *Exceptional Children, 53,* 199–208.

## BIBLIOGRAPHY/SUGGESTED READINGS

Fletcher-Janzen, E., & Reynolds, C. R. (2003). *Childhood disorders diagnostic desk reference*. Hoboken, NJ: John Wiley & Sons.

Lawson, H. (1998). *Practical record keeping: Development and resource material for staff working with pupils with special educational needs* (2nd ed.). London: D. Fulton.

Macht, J. (1998). *Special education's failed system: A question of eligibility*. Westport, CT: Bergin & Garvey.

Marzano, R. J., Pickering, D., & McTighe, J. (1993). *Assessing student outcomes: Performance assessment using the dimensions of learning model*. Alexandria, VA: Association for Supervision and Curriculum Development.

Mertens, D. M., & McLaughlin, J. A. (2004). *Research and evaluation methods in special education*. Thousand Oaks, CA: Corwin Press.

Reynolds, C. R., & Fletcher-Janzen, E. (2000). *Encyclopedia of special education: A reference for the education of the handicapped and other exceptional children and adults*. New York: J. Wiley & Sons.

Schmidt, P. R. (2005). *Preparing educators to communicate and connect with families and communities*. Greenwich, CT: Information Age Pub.

Seligman, M. (2000). *Conducting effective conferences with parents of children with disabilities: A guide for teachers*. New York: Guilford Press.

Sweeney, W. K. (1998). *The special-needs reading list: An annotated guide to the best publications for parents and professionals*. Bethesda, MD; Woodbine House.

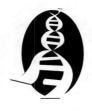

# CHAPTER 7

# The Early Years
## *Birth to 3 Programs*

*O*nce a diagnosis of VCFS is made, parents can contact their local health department for information on birth to 3 programs. Early intervention is strongly encouraged and therapy can be started at a very young age. Children should be assessed for speech and language issues and fine or gross motor delays. They also can be screened for hearing and vision difficulties.

The emphasis at this age level is to help the child reach developmental milestones with the emphasis on speech and language therapy, and remediation of fine and gross motor delays. When considering occupational therapy parents should be cautious. There is a great deal of controversy in the scientific community as to whether current therapies for sensory dysfunction are effective. One article, published in *Communique* (Shaw, 2002), argued against the effectiveness of this type of therapy, citing 41 articles that failed to scientifically prove that children improve and likened the positive effects seen by parents and therapists to a placebo effect. Another article from the same publisher (Miller, 2003) argued that there are studies suggesting the intervention works (Kinnealey, Koenig, & Huecker, 1999) and that there are flaws in Shaw's conclusions. What the authors do agree upon is that more scientific research must be gathered and the effectiveness of the treatment should be assessed using homogeneous groups of children. For example, separate tests should be conducted on children with autism, learning disabilities, attention issues, etc., and then the therapy's effectiveness can be determined. Needless to say, there are no formal studies involving children with VCFS and this therapy. Until more is known, parents will need to educate themselves and then decide if they want to pursue this treatment avenue. Some insurance companies will cover sensory integration therapy, which can be quite expensive, and others will not. A better approach would be to tailor a program to meet individual needs of the child with VCFS and not just adopt a particular therapy approach. Close monitoring on a case-by-case basis will be necessary to determine if any intervention is effective.

Parents can also work with their young child at home to improve muscle/posture strengthening, eye coordination, bilateral integration skill development, and motor planning. Closer to age 3 children can practice eye-hand coordination by coloring, catching a ball, pouring liquids, solving jigsaw puzzles, or stringing beads. Many children with VCFS have hypotonia (low muscle tone) and would benefit from strengthening exercises. Intervention to target these areas would help the child gain the necessary dexterity to be able to cut, color, and manipulate objects as he or she enters a formal school program.

## REFERENCES

Hom, E. M. (1991). Basic motor skills instruction for children with neuromotor delays: A critical review. *The Journal of Special Education*, *25*(2), 168–197.

Kinnealey, M., Koenig, K. P., & Huecker, G. E. (1999). Changes in special needs children following intensive short-term intervention. *The Journal of Developmental and Learning Disorders*, *3*, 85–103.

Miller, Lucy J. (2003). Empirical evidence related to therapies for sensory processing impairments. *NASP Communiqué*, *31*(5).

Shaw, S. R. (2002). A school psychologist investigates sensory integration therapies: Promise, possibility and the art of placebo, *NASP Communiqué*, vol. 31(2). Retrieved May, 2006 from www.nasponline.org/publications/cq/cq312index.aspx

## BIBLIOGRAPHY/SUGGESTED READINGS

Shonkoff, J., & Phillips, D. (2000). Neurons to neighborhoods: The science of early childhood development. Youth, and Families Board on Children, Committee on Integrating the Science of Early Childhood Development, National Research Council.

Stroufe, L. A. (1995). *Emotional development: The organization of emotional life in the early years*. New York: Cambridge University Press.

Tada, W. L., & Harris, S. R. (1986). *Therapeutic exercise in developmental disabilities*. Rockville, MD: Aspen Systems.

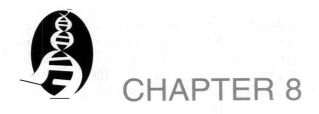

CHAPTER 8

# Getting Ready for School
## *Preschool (Ages 3–5)*

*E*ntering kindergarten can be a difficult adjustment for children with chronic health problems. Many children with VCFS have had numerous surgeries or hospitalizations before age 5 and may still suffer from fatigue, infections, feeding difficulties, and other health complications. In addition, many experience separation anxiety and will need a period of time to adjust to a new, unfamiliar environment. Planning in advance for this transition can make the adjustment easier. Preschool experiences that focus on readiness for learning activities can certainly help prepare these children for the demands of a kindergarten classroom.

Before a child is 3 years of age, parents should contact the school system and request a referral be made for special education services. In the United States children are eligible for services from age 3 to age 21 provided they meet the criteria for special education placement.

## ACCESSING SERVICES—REFERRING A CHILD FOR SPECIAL EDUCATION

Most children with VCFS will require some type of special education service as they progress from preschool through college age. The amount and depth of the needed interventions vary from child to child. Studies show a wide variation in abilities with this syndrome. Several researchers have found about 40% of the children with VCFS test in the cognitively impaired range with the majority of the rest scoring in the below average range (IQ ranging from

70 to 85). A small percentage of children have test results in the average range of intelligence. Research has also shown a tendency for IQ scores to drop with age. A theory for this decline is that the drop is due to the fact that the IQ test emphasizes abstract reasoning and higher thinking skills as a child matures. Children with VCFS tend to have a deficit in this area and that is reflected in falling test scores.

In addition to cognition deficits, children with VCFS often have speech and language delays. In the early years, intervention emphasis is often on articulation and speech sound production following pharyngeal flap surgery. Many children are quite successful with learning proper articulation and often intelligibility becomes good by kindergarten. However, as children enter school, the processing of language becomes more of an issue. Many children with VCFS test poorly in the areas of receptive and expressive language. This will impact how a child functions in a mainstreamed regular education setting.

Children with this syndrome are usually served in the U.S. public schools through the IDEA (Individuals with Disabilities Education Act) in the categories of speech and language and other health impairment. Although children with VCFS have what can be thought of as a learning disability, they often do not meet the criteria for learning disabilities as defined by special education placement criteria because there is not a large discrepancy between their IQ scores and their academic performance. Nonetheless, most will qualify for services in the areas of speech and language and/or other health impairment.

Velo-cardio-facial syndrome certainly meets the definition of other health impairment. Most children with VCFS are affected across multiple body systems that collectively impact their ability to function in class. Many are hypotonic, have reoccurring infections, attention deficits, thyroid dysfunction, heart problems, and mild hearing difficulties, and have visual/auditory processing problems. In addition, the brain research is showing medically-based abnormalities that would qualify students in this category. Finally, while many children with VCFS may also show behavioral difficulties, these problems are usually not the primary reason for their difficulty with school. If their educational needs are not properly addressed, however, they are at greater risk for developing more severe psychiatric difficulties as they mature. It is therefore imperative that educators, parents, and health professionals work together to tailor a realistic educational program that minimizes stress and fosters positive self-esteem.

Parents may refer their child for special education testing by contacting their local school district. This initial contact can be made as early as age 3 and should be done for all children diagnosed with this syndrome. Once a referral has been made, the school district must convene a special education team to evaluate the suspected area(s) of need. School districts have 90 days in which to do this evaluation, develop an education plan, and if required offer placement. Parents must give their permission for their child to be tested. Parents are a part of this team and can make suggestions regarding which areas to test. They can also provide information to the team that they have gathered through outside testing, medical reports, articles, studies, etc.

Once a child has been evaluated, the team will meet to determine if the child meets the criteria for needing special education services. This determination should be made based on norm-based test scores, classroom performance indicators, medical records, and interviews with teachers and parents. No one test (such as an IQ test) can be used as the sole determining factor as to whether a child should qualify for special education services. The team must consider several assessments to make this determination.

Children with VCFS often have many deficits that should be explored when considering special education placement. Many children with VCFS do not function well in a large group setting without reteaching or small group opportunities for learning. Although the type of program needed will vary from individual to individual, there are areas of need that seem to be shared by a great many children with this syndrome. Professionals should take a close look at these target areas when a child is referred for evaluation. The team should consider some or all of the following areas:

■ Speech and Language Needs—Articulation problems, expressive language delays, auditory processing deficits, problem-solving difficulties, reasoning difficulties, word finding problems, difficulty understanding idioms or words with multiple meanings, problems following multiple directions.

■ Learning Disability/Other Health Impairment Issues—Memory difficulties, math reasoning impairments, problems with written language elaboration, reading comprehension delays (decoding skills may be at a normal level), difficulty understanding cause and effect relationships, reasoning difficulties in social studies and science, lack of ability to apply learned knowledge to novel situations, attention and organization problems, impaired executive functioning, hypotonia (children are tired and lack stamina), fine motor coordination delays (writing, cutting, keyboarding, coloring), hearing deficits (many children have frequent ear infections or a hearing loss), physical therapy needs, lowered immune system causing frequent illnesses, vision/tracking problems, and behavioral difficulties (easily frustrated, low self-esteem, poor coping skills, difficulty getting along with peers, teased, etc.).

### IQ Measurement

Probably the most widely accepted measures of IQ are the Wechsler Intelligence Scales (WISC). There are three main types of Wechsler intelligence tests: Wechsler Preschool and Primary Scale of Intelligence (WPPSI) (ages 3–7 years), Wechsler Intelligence Scale for Children (WISC) (7–16 years), and

Wechsler Adult Intelligence Scale (WAIS) (16 years and over). The test is broken down into two sections. The verbal scale measures:

- Information: This is a measure of general knowledge.

- Digit span: Subjects are given a set of digits to repeat forwards and backwards. This is a test of immediate auditory recall and freedom from distraction.

- Vocabulary: This is a measure of expressive word knowledge.

- Arithmetic: This includes mental arithmetic and brief story type problems. It tests distractibility as well as numerical reasoning.

- Comprehension: This has questions that focus on issues of social awareness.

- Similarities: This is a measure of concept formation. Subjects are asked to say how two seemingly dissimilar items might in fact be similar.

The performance scales measure:

- Picture completion: Subjects must find a small detail in a picture that is missing.

- Picture arrangement: Subject is required to arrange pictures into a logical sequence.

- Block design: This involves putting sets of blocks together to match patterns on cards.

- Digit symbol: This involves copying a coding pattern.

- Object assembly: This includes four small jigsaw type puzzles.

There are three scores obtained from the Wechsler test: Verbal IQ, Performance IQ, and Full Scale IQ. The test can be further evaluated to identify a verbal-performance discrepancy, spatial-perception issues, and a freedom from distraction score.

Caution should be used in interpreting the test results for children with VCFS. There are so many interfering health factors that could artificially lower scores, such as poor attention abilities, vision impairments, hypotonia, fatigue, etc. It is important not to underestimate a child's potential to learn. Many children with VCFS with higher IQ measures are able to learn regular academic material with proper accommodations. It is also important to note that the IDEA law prohibits using just one score to qualify or disqualify a student for special education services.

### Speech and Language Evaluation

Several tests are available to help identify problems in the areas of speech and language. The special education team or medical professionals will be able to choose from a multitude of test instruments. It would be helpful when choosing these tests, however, if professionals are well versed in the typical profile of a child with VCFS so that they test for the commonly found areas of weakness.

## READINESS TO LEARN ACTIVITIES

Preschool education for the child with VCFS should be tailored to address deficits that occur in the areas of speech and language, sensory function, social interactions, and academic readiness. The Council on Exceptional Children recommends the following design for a preschool intervention program (Hemmeter, 2000).

This checklist centers solely on the child-focused intervention practices of the Division for Early Childhood (DEC) of the Council for Exceptional Children Recommended Practices in Early Intervention/Early Childhood Special Education (Sandall, McLean, & Smith, 2000). It does not include the DEC Recommended Practices related to assessment, teamwork, or other important aspects of early intervention/early childhood special education. Professionals can use this checklist to determine how they are doing when it comes to the delivery of instruction and support for children with disabilities. Following a period of field testing, expanded versions of this self-assessment that will include examples and non-examples of the practices will be available through DEC. This product will also cross-reference the practices with the guidelines of the National Association for the Education of Young Children (NAEYC) and the Head Start Performance Standards. Such self-assessments will be valuable as individuals, teams, and programs strive for continuous improvement. Other resources to aid in implementing the practices will include videos and training opportunities.

Adults design environments to promote children's safety, active engagement, learning, participation, and membership.

- Learning environments meet accepted standards of quality including curriculum, child-staff ratios, group size, and physical design of the classroom.

- Interventionists ensure the physical and emotional safety and security of children while children are in their care.

- A variety of appropriate settings and naturally occurring activities are used to facilitate children's learning and development.

■ Services are provided in natural learning environments as appropriate. These include places where typical children participate, such as home or community settings.

■ Physical space and materials are structured and adapted to promote engagement, play, interaction, and learning by attending to children's preferences and interests, using novelty, using responsive toys, providing adequate amounts of materials, and using defined spaces.

■ The social environment is structured to promote engagement, interaction, communication, and learning by providing peer models, peer proximity, responsive adults, imitative adults, and expanding children's play and behavior.

## Self-Assessment: Child-Focused Interventions

■ Routines and transitions are structured to promote interaction, communication, and learning by being responsive to child behavior, using naturalistic time delay, interrupted chainprocedure, transition-based teaching, and visual cue systems.

■ Play routines are structured to promote interaction, communication, and learning by defining roles for dramatic play, prompting engagement, group friendship activities, and using specialized props.

■ Environments are designed and activities are conducted so that children learn about or are exposed to multiple cultures and languages by, among other practices, allowing children and families to share their cultures and languages with others, to the extent they desire.

■ Interventionists facilitate children's engagement with their environment to encourage child-initiated learning that is not dependent on the adult's presence.

■ Adults provide environments that foster positive relationships including peer-peer, parent/caregiver-child, and parent-caregiver relationships.

Adults individualize and adapt practices for each child based on ongoing data to meet children's changing needs.

■ Practices and goals are individualized for each child based on: (a) the child's current behavior and abilities across relevant domains instead of the child's diagnostic category; (b) the family's view of what the child needs to learn; (c) interventionist and specialist views of what the child needs to learn; and (d) the demands, expectations, and requirements of the child's current environments.

■ Practices target meaningful outcomes for the child that build upon the child's current skills and behaviors and promote membership with others. Data-based decisions are used to make modifications in practices. Child performance is monitored and data are collected to determine the impact of the practices on the child's progress and to make modifications in the intervention if needed. The ongoing monitoring must be feasible and useful within the child's environment.

■ Recommended practices are used to teach/promote whatever skills are necessary for children to function more completely, competently, adaptively, and independently in the child's natural environments. These skills should be those that maximize participation and membership in home, school, and community environments, including those that are typical or similar to other persons' in those environments. Attention should be given to the breadth and sophistication of the child's skills.

■ Children's behavior is recognized, interpreted in context, responded to contingently, and opportunities are provided for expansion or elaboration of child behavior by imitating the behavior, waiting for the child's responses, modeling, and prompting.

Adults use systematic procedures within and across environments, activities, and routines to promote children's learning and participation.

■ Interventionists are agents of change to promote and accelerate learning, and that learning should be viewed in different phases (i.e., acquisition, fluency, maintenance, generalization) that require different types of practices.

■ Practices are used systematically, frequently, and consistently within and across environments (e.g., home, center, community) and across people (i.e., those who care for and interact regularly with the child).

■ Planning that considers the situation (e.g., class, home, etc.) in which the intervention will be applied occurs prior to implementation.

■ Practices that are used are validated, normalized, useful across environments, respectful, and not stigmatizing of the child and family and are sensitive to linguistic and cultural issues.

■ Systematic naturalistic teaching procedures such as models, expansions, incidental teaching, Peer-mediated strategies are used to promote social and communicative behavior.

■ Prompting and fading procedures (e.g., modeling, graduated guidance, increasing assistance, time delay) are used to ensure acquisition and use of communicative, self-care, cognitive, and social skills.

■ Instructional strategies such as those described above are embedded and distributed within and across activities.

■ Recommended instructional strategies are used with sufficient fidelity, consistency, frequency, and intensity to ensure high levels of behavior occurring frequently.

■ Consequences for children's behavior are structured to increase the complexity and duration of children's play, engagement, appropriate behavior, and learning by using differential reinforcement, response shaping, high-probability procedures (i.e., behavioral momentum), and correspondence training.

■ For problem behaviors, interventionists should assess the behavior in context to identify its function, and then devise interventions that are comprehensive in that they make the behavior irrelevant (i.e., the child's environment is modified so that problem behavior is unnecessary or precluded), inefficient (i.e., a more efficient replacement behavior is taught), and ineffective (i.e., reinforcement and other consequent events are used).

With these guidelines in mind, a preschool program for VCFS children should include several specific interventions. As mentioned earlier, a large percentage of children with VCFS will need speech therapy to learn correct muscle control in their mouths. This therapy should be occurring during this time. At preschool children can receive direct services to work on articulation, pragmatic speech, and understanding language.

Children with VCFS often struggle at this time with intelligibility. This can be frustrating both for the children who are desperately trying to communicate and the caretakers who are struggling to understand them. Patience, flexibility, and frequent positive reinforcement seem to help. Children with VCFS learn best by repetition and modeling. They also need frequent reinforcement for correct speech and respond well to games and behavioral modification approaches.

Care should also be taken to encourage positive social relationships with peers. Teasing is a problem for many children with VCFS because they may sound different from others. They may also have poor oral muscle control that for some can lead to unintended drooling. Subtle cues by the teacher can help eliminate this, as can muscle strengthening exercises. In the meantime, however, adults should monitor social interactions and help the child with VCFS understand the language needed for play and friendship. Role playing, social playgroups, and social stories all help provide the needed practice to enhance language skills.

In addition, occupational therapy may still be indicated to address areas of sensory dysfunction. At preschool, teachers must be informed as to the nature of the problem so that accommodations can be made to the environment. That could include simplifying the environment to reduce sensory overload, providing a spot where the child feels comfortable and safe, giving preferential seating near the teacher, controlling auditory distractions like buzzing bulbs or noisy aquariums, providing headphones and calming music during quiet times, and providing comfortable seating.

Children with VCFS also need a consistent routine that is predictable. Posted schedules, organized supplies and toys, and structure to the day help them keep calm and on track. They will also need a great deal of help organizing their own supplies and belongings. Having a plan for where they can place their supplies, coats, backpacks, and lunch will help, but they will need this behavior modeled and repeated. They also may need support for manipulating these because of low muscle tone and difficulty with dressing, etc. They also will need more time do accomplish tasks and to process information. Build this extra needed time into their routine.

In addition, transitions need to be carefully planned. Children with VCFS need plenty of notice that an activity will change. Cues should be both verbal and visual such as posting a picture of food on a magnetic board before snack time along with saying, "In five minutes we will be cleaning up for snack time." Some teachers use music to signify a transition or jingle a bell. If the child is fidgety, provide opportunities for movement during transition time.

Children with VCFS learn best by doing. Multiple opportunities to practice and model skills work best. They will retain very little of what is said in a large group setting and will need one-on-one or small group experiences to grasp concepts. Thus, if the idea of the calendar is presented in a large setting, give children with VCFS their own calendar to color or decorate. Have them count days with an adult and perhaps paste the names of the days in the proper places. Have them verbally retell what they understand, reinforce, and practice the skill multiple times. Drill and practice is particularly helpful for mastery of skills. Make instructions simple and uncomplicated. Recognize that more adult help will be needed for a child with VCFS to complete a task than may be needed for others in the class.

Finally, keep a calm and quiet voice level. A loud voice will be misinterpreted as an angry voice. Whispering can be more effective than a loud, forceful tone. Expectations should be realistic, but children with VCFS should be taught at a typical preschool level. Many can grasp the concepts, learn to sight-read words, and learn to count at an appropriate level. They should also learn proper school behavior expectations so they can move on to kindergarten and function in a school environment. These readiness skills are necessary for successful movement to a public school classroom.

## INTENSIVE MATH READINESS INSTRUCTION

As discussed in earlier chapters, the research done involving children with VCFS suggests that most will have significant difficulty with math concepts. It is prudent, therefore, to be proactive and begin math remediation as early as possible. Although a lot of research has been done on the field of language/ reading disabilities, there are far fewer studies on remedial programs for math.

A math disability (or dyscalculia) is an individual's difficulty in conceptualizing numbers, numerical relationships, estimation, and numerical operations (Sharma, 2003). It can be quantitative, which relates more to counting and calculating and quannitative, which involves trouble understanding math processes, spatial relationships, and the concepts of time, space, and quantity.

Persons with dyscalculia have trouble with:

- Mastering facts by the usual methods, especially those involving counting.

- Dealing with situations involving money, bank accounts, budgeting, etc.

- Understanding the abstract concepts of time or the sequencing of events.

- Conceptualizing spatial orientation, directionality, left/right orientation reading maps.

- Following sequential direction, organization, reversing numbers, and remembering specific facts.

Early intervention to address these deficits should include intensive exposure to activities that help the child gain number sense. Sharma breaks math readiness into the following seven prerequisite skills (Sharma, 2003):

- The ability to follow sequential directions

- A keen sense of directionality, of one's position in space, of spatial orientation and space organization; examples include the ability to tell left from right, north/south/east/west, up/down/, forward/ backward

- Pattern recognition and its extension

- Visualization: the ability to conjure up pictures in one's mind and manipulate them

- Estimation: the ability to form a reasonable educated guess about size, amount, number, and magnitude

- Deductive reasoning: the ability to reason from the general principle to a particular instance, or reasoning from a stated premise to a logical conclusion

- Inductive reasoning: a natural understanding that is not the result of conscious attention or reasoning, easily seeing the patterns in different situations and the interrelationships between procedures and concepts

Before children can begin to understand factual operations, such as adding and subtraction, they need to have a solid grasp of these math-readiness skills. Otherwise, they will not really understand the math concepts behind the operations or have the math foundation upon which to build more abstract ideas. In addition, they must understand the language of math terminology. The linguistic elements of math language should be directly taught. Concrete examples, field trips, and experiments can all be used to help the child conceptualize the math ideas. Constructing a model or demonstrating the math concept with manipulatives will help the child visualize and remember the concept. The use of a number line and a thermometer can be a useful way to try to demonstrate numerical relationships. Teachers should also keep in mind the research results out of Simon's lab regarding students with VCFS and deficits in magnitude recognition. Since many children with VCFS have difficulty recognizing subtle differences in quantities, examples for early learning should emphasize larger, more obvious differences. As the child becomes more skilled, harder, less obvious problems can be introduced. Try to relate the learning to meaningful experiences that directly apply to the child. For example, relate the idea to the child's own family or a situation in the classroom.

A new McGraw-Hill/SRA program (available through http://www.SRA online.com) called Number Worlds specifically targets math readiness skills. It is designed for students who show difficulty mastering math concepts and who are functioning below expected grade level. The company designed part of its program to be preventative in nature and for use with preschool and kindergarten-age children. The program is new on the market, so independent, evidenced-based data are not available on its effectiveness. However, considering the research on math difficulties associated with VCFS, it might be worth exploring.

The Number Worlds program at this level can be used as a whole class program or in a resource room setting, after school, or in summer school. It combines hands-on opportunities with computer learning, discussion, and paper-pencil activities so multiple modalities are available to present the concepts. In the preschool/kindergarten levels, students acquire counting and quality schemas, develop a core conceptual understanding of single-digit numbers, and then link this understanding to a formal symbol system. It helps form intuition and number sense, the basis for future success with mathematical computation and reasoning. The Building Blocks computer software component of the program adds more opportunities to practice the skills with visual and auditory feedback. The use of the computer was shown to be an effective approach to teaching children with VCFS, so this aspect of this program may be particularly useful (Kok & Solman, 1995). The SRA company cites research funded by the National Science Foundation that supports use of this program with students who are struggling with math.

The On Cloud Nine math program is another attempt to remediate math difficulties through the use of early intervention strategies. This program is available through the Lindamood-Bell Learning Company (http://www.linda

moodbell.com).The program moves though three basic steps to develop mathematical reasoning and computation. The first is the use of manipulatives to experience the realness of math, the second is imagery and language to concretize that reality in the sensory system, and third is to apply computation skills to problem-solving situations. The program is based on the theory that math is thinking (dual coding), with imagery, and language. In other words, to understand math one must be able to mentally "picture" or see its logic (Bell & Tuley, 2006). Dual coding requires two aspects in imagery: symbol/numeral imagery (parts/details) and concept imagery (whole/gestalt). Visualizing numbers is one of the basic cognitive processes needed for math understanding. Activities are included that teach number preservation (the concept that the number 5 represents a set of five things), the visualization of chronological relationships (such as a number line, days of the week), and the use of imagery to compute and conceptualize math.

At home, parents can help their children acquire number sense by asking them to ascend and count four steps and then count and descend two steps. They can use thermometers, elevators, etc., to teach the concept of numbers going up and down. They can also use activities such as setting the table for the correct number of persons in the family to reinforce the concept of one-to-one correspondence. Finally, children will benefit from verbalizing how they are attempting to solve a math problem. Talking about math strategies will help reinforce basic concepts and will lead to deeper understanding of numbers.

A third possible intervention that can be considered is the pre-school program through the Singapore Math Company. The Web site http://www.singaporemath.com has sample pages and explanations concerning the curriculum. The Singapore students consistently lead the world in mathematics, and preliminary studies with students using this curriculum in the United States are promising. The drawback, as with any of the other interventions, is that there are no formal studies showing success with students who have VCFS. However, in looking at the program, there are reasons to believe that this would be a good match for children with VCFS. First, the pages in the workbooks are relatively clean and uncluttered. This is a good format for the students visually. Concepts are also presented pictorially and with words. Second, the philosophy of the program is to reduce the content in the curriculum. Students work for mastery of a concept rather than learn incrementally with a spiral approach. Concepts are not repeated year after year, but rather covered in depth at age-appropriate levels. This philosophy, which encourages depth rather than breadth, allows struggling students multiple opportunities within a time period to digest the information. Finally, a large emphasis of the program is to teach strategies for solving problems. For example, the program teaches several strategies to understand the concept of subtraction. Students also verbalize how they are attempting to solve problems. This discussion fosters deeper understanding and mastery.

## PHONEMIC AWARENESS INSTRUCTION

Current research into reading success is pointing to phonemic awareness as one of the best predictors of how well students will learn to read during the first two years of school (Vaugh & Linan-Thompson, 2004). Phonemic awareness is the ability to segment words into their very basic sounds. For example, the word *bat* has three separate phonemes: /b/, /a/, and /t/. It is also the ability to blend sounds, rhyme words, and manipulate sounds to make new words. Phonological awareness skills and activities can include the following:

- Discriminating—Students listen to words to determine if they have the same beginning sounds.

- Counting—Students clap the number of words in a sentence.

- Rhyming—Students make word families with rhyming words (hit, lit, bit. sit).

- Alliteration—Students create tongue twisters using words with the same first letter sound (She sells sea shells by the seashore).

- Blending—Students say the individual sounds in the word and then say them quickly to blend sounds.

- Segmenting—Students break words into syllables.

- Manipulating—Students add, delete, or substitute sounds and syllables in words.

Explicit instruction in these phonemic skills would benefit the child with VCFS and would help lay the foundation for beginning literary skills. Some of this instruction can occur in a preschool classroom or during speech and language therapy. It is important to keep in mind that many children with VCFS have recurring ear infections and some have intermittent mild hearing loss. Early attention to hearing sounds is important to make sure that beginning listening skills are adequately addressed. Decoding words is a relative strength for many VCFS beginning readers. This may, in part, be due to the intensive speech therapy many of them receive at an early age.

## HANDLING BEHAVIOR ISSUES

Many children with VCFS suffer from separation anxiety at a young age. Often these children have had several surgeries and they do not process sensory input well. Patience and understanding are needed to help the child feel safe and comfortable in a new setting. Parents can help by preparing their child for the day by talking about the school and the day's scheduled activities. It is often best for parents to leave, even if the child is crying, so that the staff can take over and redirect the child to a favorite activity. It may be necessary to assign a particular staff member to greet the child as he or she arrives, so that there is some consistency in the first school interaction of the day. In severe cases, it may be necessary to seek the assistance of a professional to deal with this issue.

Children with VCFS often are diagnosed with attention deficits. Using strategies that work for children with ADD may produce some success, but usually more is needed. It is best to keep the verbal instructions to a minimum. A long drawn-out explanation will likely not be understood. Keep directions short and model appropriate behavior. Realize that most children with VCFS will not easily generalize classroom rules to new situations. Many will need repeated reminders and multiple practice opportunities. Do not expect these children to be able to verbally explain what happened in a situation or to say what they should have done differently. Do not expect them to problem-solve easily or to fully understand logical consequences. Rather use modeling, verbal cues, rewards, and foreshadowing of transitions to help with behavior. Learning to behave in school is an important concept for future success, so early intervention for behavior problems is imperative. For additional behavior intervention ideas see Appendix A.

## REFERENCES

Bell, N., & Tuley, K. (2006). *Imagery: The sensory-cognitive connection for math*. Learning Disabilities Online. Retrieved from http://www.ldonline.org/indepth.

Kok, L. L., & Solman, R. T. (1995). Velocardiofacial syndrome: Learning difficulties and intervention. *Journal of Medical Genetics, 32*(8), 612–618.

Sandall, S., McLean, M. E., & Smith, B. J. (2000). *DEC recommended practices in early intervention/early childhood special education*. Longmont, CO: Sopris West.

Sharma, M. (2003). *Dyslexia, dyscalculia, remediation: Math notebooks*. Berkshire Mathematics. Retrieved 2006 from http://www.berkshiremamatics.com.

Vaughn, S., & Linan-Thompson, S. (2004). *Research-based methods of reading instruction*. Alexandria, VA: Association for Supervision and Curriculum Development.

## BIBLIOGRAPHY/SUGGESTED READINGS

Beaty, J. J. (1992). *Skills for preschool teachers*. New York: M. Macmillan International.

Brazelton, T. B., & Greenspan, S. I. (2000). *The irreducible needs of children: What every child must have to grow, learn, and flourish*. Cambridge, MA: Perseus.

Catron, C. E., & Allen, J. (1993). *Early childhood curriculum*. New York; Toronto: Merrill; Maxwell Macmillan Canada.

Dixon, T. (1990). *Jessica and the wolf: A story for children who have bad dreams*. Washington, DC: Magination Press.

Dutro, J. (1991). *Night light: A story for children afraid of the dark*. Washington, DC: Magination Press.

Gould, P., & Sullivan, S. (2005). *The Inclusive early childhood classroom: Easy ways to adapt learning centers for all*. Prentice Hall.

Gutstein, S. E., & Sheely, R. K. (2002). *Relationship development intervention with young children: Social and emotional development activities for Asperger syndrome, autism, PDD, and NLD*. London; Philadelphia: Jessica Kingsley.

Hendrick, J. (1992). *The whole child: Developmental education for the early years*. New York; Toronto: Merrill; Maxwell Macmillan Canada; Maxwell Macmillan International.

Kostelnik, M. J. (2002). *Children with special needs: Lessons for early childhood professionals*. New York: Teachers College Press.

Kostelnik, Soderman, & Whiren. (2004). *Developmentally appropriate curriculum: Best practices in early childhood education*. Prentice-Hall.

Marcus, I. W., Marcus, P., & Jeschke, S. (1992). *Into the Great forest: A story for children leaving home for the first time*. Washington, DC: Magination Press.

Read, K. H., Gardner, P., & Mahler, B. C. (1993). *Early childhood programs: Human relationships and learning*. Fort Worth, TX: Harcourt Brace Jovanovich College Publishers.

Silverman, W. K., & Ollendick, T. H. (1999). *Developmental issues in the clinical treatment of children*. Boston: Allyn and Bacon.

Sroufe, L. A. (1995). *Emotional development:The organization of emotional life in the early years*. New York: Cambridge University Press.

Wolery, M., & Wilbers, J. S. (1994). *Including children with special needs in early childhood programs*. Washington, DC: National Association for the Education of Young Children.

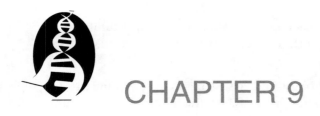

## CHAPTER 9

# Entering a Formal School Education Program

$M$any parents struggle to find the right fit for their child with developmental disabilities. While the emphasis in this book is on educating a child within the parameters of a public school program, it is worth noting that some parents choose to school their child at home or at a private school setting. This decision is often a very difficult one for families, from both a time and expense standpoint.

There are several points to consider when deciding whether to opt for a less traditional approach to education. Some issues when thinking about home schooling or a private school are:

- Will the removal of the child from the public school limit access to educational materials and current curriculum resources (examples: science labs, computer equipment, textbook resources)?

- Will the child have access to an educator trained to teach using techniques for students with learning difficulties?

- Will speech, occupational, physical therapy services be available to the child?

- Will the child develop the necessary skills for independently functioning in a school setting (examples: study skills, time management, independent work habits, etc.)?

- Will he or she be exposed to normally developing peers for friendships and role modeling?

■ Will the private school placement or home offer opportunities for specialized training in art, music, consumer education, career exploration, and job skills?

■ Will there be accountability and assessments given regularly to insure adequate academic progress? Is the alternative program appropriately challenging?

Clearly, there are many questions to answer. The ultimate long-term goal to keep in mind is what the family's realistic dream is for the future. At the very least, it is hoped that the child will graduate with skills necessary for a job, will maintain a preserved self concept, will acquire social skills needed to support a happy, connected adult life, and will have many skills necessary for independent living outside of the parent's home. In addition, many parents hope that the young adult will be able to participate in a post-secondary training program or college to improve their child's opportunity for a better paying job. This is a realistic goal for some students with VCFS and should be carefully considered when planning an academic program. It might be best to program with the hope this is attainable and then adjust the academic program later if needed. With medical advancements in treating cognitive disabilities, there are many reasons to believe that a bright future lies ahead. Whatever school placement is decided upon, using the accommodations suggested in this book will help insure a quality education and learning success.

## CLASSROOM ENVIRONMENT

Ideally the classroom environment for a child with VCFS should be inviting, yet uncluttered. As mentioned earlier, one area of deficit in the population is in the area of visual processing. An environment that is cluttered, with many distracting pictures and signs, will make it difficult for the child to locate materials. The room should also be organized with important areas clearly marked. Many children with VCFS learn to read words relatively easily so written signs with large, simple print can help. They also should have their desks situated close to the front of the room.

Some schools are using some different technology to replace the typical chalkboard or whiteboard. A Smart Board is an innovative system that melds computer capabilities with a whiteboard. A finger or pen can be used directly on the screen to write, erase, or perform mouse functions. Students can become physically involved with the presentation by writing on the board or dragging icons across the screen. The screen is large, so students with visual/spatial deficits have an easier time reading the font. Another advantage of this system over the typical classroom chalkboard is the ability to add a visual component to presentations. For example, the class can read a paragraph on the screen and then click to view a video clip of the subject matter. This capability has endless applications and the benefit of enhancing comprehension of written matter. The system also has math software that can be purchased to help illustrate abstract math concepts in a concrete fashion (Figure 9–1). Information about the board is available at http://www.smarttech.com.

There also should be an effort to minimize extra noise. Many children with VCFS have a mild hearing loss or frequent ear infections. Their hearing can fluctuate from day to day. Some children benefit from using an FM system. An FM system has two components. The teacher wears a mini-microphone and the child wears a receiving earpiece. The teacher's voice is amplified and becomes the dominant sound the child hears. This can help with focus and concentration because other competing classroom noises are minimized. The drawback, however, is that with older models during discussions the microphone needs to be passed to others around the room for the system to be effective. Newer systems eliminate this problem by using a room amplifier. Even with the older system's limitations, the use of an FM can be helpful to a child with hearing difficulty. The system has also been used successfully with students who have attention issues, with no hearing loss.

The school should also assign a staff member to serve as the child's case manager. This person will oversee the student's progress, monitor implementation of necessary accommodations, and be a liaison between parents and teachers. Many students with VCFS respond very well to adults and they welcome this interaction. A staff member to help them to negotiate through school on day-to-day basis is a necessary part of their program from kindergarten through college. Although this person may change each year, it is very important

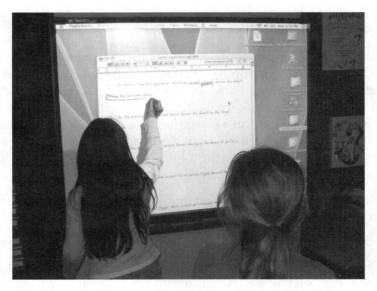

**FIGURE 9–1.** Student using the interactive Smart Board.

that the child with VCFS has a particular staff member (in addition to the regular classroom teacher) who will have time to assist this student on a one-to-one basis, serve as an advocate, and communicate regularly with parents. Furthermore, having a friendly staff member to help solve problems will lessen the student's anxiety and will make school a more positive experience.

## SENSORY INTEGRATION PROGRAM

As stated in earlier chapters, children with VCFS are often diagnosed with attention difficulties and have trouble with self-regulation. Schools can help in these areas by instituting schoolwide programs that help teach self-monitoring skills. One such program, entitled How Does Your Engine Run? The Alert Program for Self Regulation by Mary Sue Williams and Sherry Shellenberger (Williams & Shellenberger, 1996), has been successfully implemented in the United States. It is for use by occupational therapists, teachers, parents, and other professionals. The program teaches students to become aware of their arousal states and show them how to regulate themselves through the use of sensorimotor strategies. This, in turn, helps students manage their levels of alertness to learn more efficiently and to interact more appropriately within the school environment. Students first learn to rate themselves on a high-low chart (high—overstimulated to just right to low—lethargic). They do this several times throughout the school day. Next, they learn how to change their "engine levels" by using an appropriate sensorimotor strategy. These strategies are custom tailored to the student's needs and include the following methods:

- Oral input: put something in mouth (example: eat, chew gum, blow, suck)

- Vestibular and proprioceptive inputs: move through oscillation (up and down such as jumping, teeter-totter, bouncing on a therapy ball), linear (front and back such as swinging, rocking in a chair), rotary (circles such as merry-go-round or twirling), inverted (upside down such as hanging on a playground bar or walking wheelbarrow fashion), doing heavy muscular work such as pushing furniture, pulling a sled, or "crashing and bumping" such as jumping into a pile of pillows or playing bumper cars

- Touch: e.g., hold objects, squeeze a ball, snuggle under a blanket, pet an animal, play with clay, etc.

- Look: change natural lighting (dim versus bright, bold color versus pastel)

- Listen: e.g., vary noise level, listen to music, change rhythm, limit auditory distraction

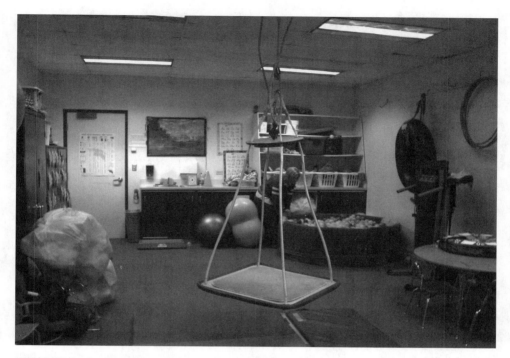

**FIGURE 9–2.** Sensory room in an elementary school where students can go to settle down and refocus.

Some schools designate a particular room where students can go when they need to apply one of the more physical strategies (Figure 9–2). Most of these methods, however, can take place in the regular classroom with minimal disruption to normal classroom routine. As the child matures, these self-regulation techniques can be used discreetly between classes, at lunch, or during class without teacher involvement.

The next several chapters discuss concerns and interventions according to age level. In programming for an older child, it is recommended that you read the suggestions for younger students in addition to those presented for the child's current school placement. Many accommodations are not age specific, and understanding earlier learning strategies with deepen an overall grasp of the syndrome. Moreover, some students may benefit from interventions suggested for earlier age levels if their skills are below an age-appropriate level.

## REFERENCES

Williams, M., & Shellenberger, S. (1996). *How does your engine run? A leader's guide to the Alert Program for Self-Regulation*. Albuquerque, NM: Therapy Works.

## BIBLIOGRAPHY/SUGGESTED READINGS

Armstrong, T. (1999). *ADD/ADHD alternatives in the classroom*. Alexandria, VA: Association for Supervision and Curriculum Development.

Armstrong, T., & Association for Supervision and Curriculum Development. (2000). *Multiple intelligences in the classroom*. Alexandria, VA: Association for Supervision and Curriculum Development.

Bender, W. N. (2002). *Differentiating instruction for students with learning disabilities: Best teaching practices for general and special educators*. Thousand Oaks, CA: Corwin Press; Council for Exceptional Children.

Benton, P., & O'Brien, T. (2000). *Special needs and the beginning teacher*. New York, NY: Continuum.

Blenk, K., & Fine, D. R. (1995). *Making school inclusion work: A guide to everyday practice*. Cambridge, MA: Brookline Books.

Byrnes, J. P. (2001). *Minds, brains, and learning: Understanding the psychological and educational relevance of neuroscientific research*. New York: Guilford Press.

Council for Exceptional Children. (2005). *What every special educator must know: Ethics, standards, and guidelines for special educators* (special 5th ed.). Upper Saddle River, NJ: Pearson/Merrill/Prentice Hall.

Crockett, J. B., & Kauffman, J. M. (1999). *The least restrictive environment: Its origins and interpretations in special education*. Mahwah, NJ: L. Erlbaum Associates.

Cunningham, C., & Davis, H. (1985). *Working with parents: Frameworks for collaboration*. Philadelphia: Open University Press.

Dover, W. (1994). *The inclusion facilitator*. Manhattan, KS: The Master Teacher Inc.

Dowdy, C. A. (1998). *Attention-deficit/hyperactivity disorder in the classroom: A practical guide for teachers*. Austin, TX: Pro-Ed.

Fink, D. B. (2000). *Making a place for kids with disabilities*. Westport, CT: Praeger.

Friend, M. P., & Bursuck, W. D. (1999). *Including students with special needs: A practical guide for classroom teachers*. Boston: Allyn and Bacon.

Goodman, G. (1994). *Inclusive classrooms from A to Z: A handbook for educators*. Columbus, OH: Teachers Publishing Group.

Kugelmass, J. W. (2004). *The inclusive school: Sustaining equity and standards*. New York: Teachers College Press.

LaForge, A. E. (1999). *What really happens in school: A guide to your child's emotional, social, and intellectual development, Grades K–5*. New York: Hyperion.

Lehmann, K. J. (2004). *Surviving inclusion*. Lanham, MD: Scarecrow Education.

Mather, N., & Goldstein, S. (2001). *Learning disabilities and challenging behaviors: A guide to intervention and classroom management*. Baltimore: P. H. Brookes.

Mazurek, K., & Winzer, M. A. (2000). *Special education in the 21st century: Issues of inclusion and reform*. Washington DC: Gallaudet University Press.

McCabe, M. E. (1989). *The nurturing classroom: Developing self-esteem, thinking skills, and responsibility through simple cooperation*. Willits, CA: ITA Publications.

McDonnell, L., McLaughlin, M. J., & Morison, P. (1997). *Educating one and all: Students with disabilities and standards-based reform*. Washington, DC: National Academy Press.

Pfeiffer, S. I., & Reddy, L. A. (1999). *Inclusion practices with special needs students: Theory, research, and application*. New York: Haworth Press.

Rief, S. F., & Heimburge, J. A. (1996). *How to reach and teach all students in the inclusive classroom: Ready-to-use strategies, lessons, and activities for teaching students with diverse learning needs.* West Nyack, NY: Center for Applied Research in Education.

Rourke, B. (1989). *Nonverbal learning disabilities: The syndrome and the model.* New York: The Guilford Press.

Rourke, B. (1995). *Syndrome of nonverbal learning disabilities: Neurodevelopmental manifestations.* New York, NY: The Guilford Press.

Schwartz, D. (2005). *Including children with special needs: A handbook for educators and parents.* Westport, CT: Greenwood Press.

Stainback, S. B., Stainback, W. C., & Forest, M. (1989). *Educating all students in the mainstream of regular education.* Baltimore: P. H. Brookes.

Tanquay, P., & Thompson, S. (2002). *Nonverbal learning disabilities at school: Educating students with NLD, Asperger syndrome and related conditions.* London: Jessica Kingsley.

Thompson, S. (1997). *The source for non-verbal learning disorders.* East Moline, IL: LinguiSystems.

Villa, R. A., & Thousand, J. S. (2005). *Creating an inclusive school* (2nd ed.). Alexandria, VA: Association for Supervision and Curriculum Development.

Vitello, S. J., & Mithaug, D. E. (1998). *Inclusive schooling: National and international perspectives.* Mahwah, NJ: L. Erlbaum Associates.

Wade, S. E. (2000). *Inclusive education: A casebook and readings for prospective and practicing teachers.* Mahwah, NJ: L. Erlbaum Associates.

Winebrenner, S., & Espeland, P. (1996). *Teaching kids with learning difficulties in the regular classroom: Strategies and techniques every teacher can use to challenge and motivate struggling students.* Minneapolis, MN: Free Spirit Publishing.

Woodward, J., & Cuban, L. (2001). *Technology, curriculum, and professional development: Adapting schools to meet the needs of students with disabilities.* Thousand Oaks, CA: Corwin Press.

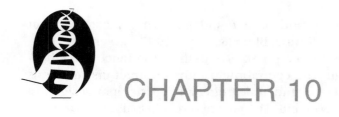

# CHAPTER 10

# Building the Foundation

## *Kindergarten through Second Grade (Ages 5–7)*

*C*hildren with velo-cardio-facial syndrome often can function in a regular education classroom with resource support. Some students also require an aide in the classroom to help them keep focused and to clarify steps and directions. Educators should keep in mind that the learning profiles of children with this syndrome vary and that many factors influence how a particular child will progress in school. However, awareness that the pattern of strengths and weaknesses seem to hold true for a large number of children with VCFS will help teachers respond quickly if difficulties develop. With this in mind, there are educational approaches that are best practice strategies for teaching most students with this syndrome.

In general, most children with VCFS have strengths in the areas of rote memorization, spelling, decoding, creative writing, and music. Deficits are usually seen in the areas of reading comprehension, math applications, problem solving, analyzing content, remembering complex information, and higher order thinking skills.

Direct instruction is one specific model of teacher-directed explicit instruction that has shown to be effective with learning disabled students. A recent review of 34 research studies comparing direct instruction (DI) interventions to a variety of other instructional programs showed that 87% of the post-treatment gains favored DI compared to only 12% that favored non-DI approaches, and 64% of statistically significant outcomes supported DI, compared to only 1% that favored non-DI approaches and 35% that favored neither. (Adams & Engelmann, 1996). Other studies have also analyzed effective intervention programs in special education and have found positive results for direct instruction methods (Forness, Kavale, Blum, & Lloyd, 1997; Tarver, 1999).

The direct instruction model emphasizes both the importance of methodology and curriculum design. The central philosophy of direct instruction is that teachers are responsible for student learning and curriculum design is a critical piece of student achievement. The goal of direct instruction is to maximize efficiency in learning. This is especially important for children with VCFS who tire easily, have difficulty focusing, and have memory difficulties. Efficiency is reached when students are able to generalize the content beyond the specific material in the lesson. During direct instruction, generalizations can be taught explicitly by using examples and non-examples to help students understand the critical elements necessary for a generalization to occur. The ability to generalize is difficult for students with VCFS, so programs to address this issue would be very helpful. There are many specific DI programs published for teaching the academic subjects at the elementary level. More information about these programs can be found at the Association for Direct Instruction at http://www.adihome.org.

## READING

In 1997, Congress asked the Director of the National Institute of Child Health and Human Development (NICHD) at the National Institutes of Health, in consultation with the Secretary of Education, to convene a national panel to assess the effectiveness of different approaches used to teach children to read.

For over two years, the National Reading Panel in the United States analyzed thousands of citations for research methodology and determined several components that enhance reading instruction (www.nichd.nih.gov/research/supported/nrp.cfm) Here is a summary of their report published in 2000 (National Reading Panel, 2000).

In the area of alphabetics, the first recommendation is instruction in phonemic awareness (PA). Phonemic awareness involves teaching children to focus on and manipulate phonemes in spoken syllables and words. (This is not the same as phonics instruction, which teaches students to use letter-sound relations to read or spell words, or auditory discrimination, which refers to the ability to recognize whether two spoken words are the same or different). Phonemic awareness involves the ability to identify phonemes, the smallest identified unit of sound that makes a difference in the spoken word. Children can manipulate phonemes to blend sounds and rhyme words. After reviewing close to 2,000 citations and identifying 52 that satisfied the National Research Panel's criteria for research methodology, it determined that teaching children to manipulate phonemes in words was highly effective under a variety of teaching conditions and grade levels. The panel found that the most effective programs provided explicit instruction in phonemic awareness and worked with children in small groups. Children who enter school with little phonetic awareness have trouble acquiring alphabetic coding skill and thus have difficulty recognizing words (Stanovich, 2000) Several tests can be used to determine if students need additional help with phonemic awareness and are also useful for monitoring progress. They are:

- Test of Phonological Awareness (TOPA; Torgesen & Bryant, 1994)
- Comprehensive Test of Phonological Processing (CTOPP; Wagner, Torgesen, & Rasholte, 1999)
- Yopp-Singer Test of Phoneme Segmentation (Yopp, 1995)
- Phoneme Segmentation Fluency (Dynamic Indicators of Basic Early Literacy Skills [DIBELS]; Kaminski & Good, 1996)

Second, the panel looked at phonics instruction. The primary purpose of teaching phonics is to help children understand how letters are linked to sounds (phonemes) to form letter-sound relationships and spelling patterns. The panel found that teaching phonics produced significant benefits for students in kindergarten through sixth grade and also improved the reading scores of students having difficulty learning to read. It also found that explicit, systematic phonics instruction was significantly more effective than instruction that teaches little or no phonics. The panel cautioned that learning letter sounds was not an end in itself and that children must be able to apply this knowledge to their daily reading and writing activities.

The panel also looked at the area of fluency or the ability to read orally with speed, accuracy, and proper expression. Fluency is a necessary component of reading comprehension but is often overlooked in the classroom. The panel found the instructional method of guided oral reading (where the student receives systematic and explicit feedback and guidance from an adult) had a significant and positive impact on word recognition, fluency, and comprehension across grade levels. It also looked at independent silent reading as a method to increase student reading achievement. Although there have been many studies that show a correlation between time spent reading and reading achievement, the panel was unable to find a scientifically sound positive relationship between programs and instruction that encourage large amounts of independent reading with minimal guidance or feedback and improvements in reading achievement or fluency. The positive correlation found in many studies, they conclude, may be more due to the fact that children who are proficient in reading enjoy it and thus read more.

Finally, in the area of comprehension, which is of greatest concern for students with VCFS, the panel had several suggestions. First, vocabulary instruction does lead to gains in comprehension, but it must be appropriate for the student's ability. Vocabulary instruction using computers is a promising tool and is emerging as a valuable aid to teachers. Second, students should be taught to use specific cognitive strategies or to reason strategically when they encounter confusing text. The panel found seven categories of compre-hension instruction that are effective based on scientific studies for non-impaired readers. They are:

- Comprehension monitoring—where readers learn how to judge whether they understand the material

- Cooperative learning—where students learn reading strategies together

- Use of graphic and semantic organizers (including story maps) to make pictorial representations of the material to assist with under-standing

- Question answering—where readers answer questions posed by the teacher and get immediate feedback

- Question generation—where readers ask themselves questions about various aspects of the story

- Story structure—where students are taught to use the structure of the story as a means of helping them recall story content in order to answer questions about what they have read

- Summarization—where readers are taught to integrate ideas and generalize from the text information

The report did not discuss whether studies of these instructional strategies have shown successful outcomes for disabled readers.

Finally, the panel looked at the use of computer technology and reading instruction. New computers, with speech recognition capabilities and advanced multimedia functions, are opening more possibilities into reading instruction. Although there were only 21 studies found that met the panel's research methodology criteria, the results are positive. In addition, the use of hyper-text (highlighted text that links to underlying definitions or related text) and the use of computers as word processors also show promise in enhancing reading and writing instruction.

An excellent source for primary teachers giving specific instructions for teaching reading is *Research-Based Methods of Reading Instruction, Grades K-3* (Vaughn & Linan-Thompson, 2004). This book looks at the National Reading Panel's recommendations and gives specific activities to target the areas of phonemic awareness, phonics, fluency, vocabulary, and comprehen-sion. Although the book is targeted for grades K-3, it is also a useful reference for upper elementary teachers, especially in the areas of fluency and com-prehension. Another book, Strategies that Work (Harvey & Goudvis, 2000), targets reading comprehension and offers helpful suggestions for teaching the concepts of making connections, questioning, visualizing, inferring, deter-mining importance and synthesizing.

Most students with VCFS can learn to read using a sight vocabulary combined with a phonemic awareness and phonics-based approach. A well-structured reading program with direct instruction on skills is preferable and many, such as those from the SRA-McGraw-Hill Company, have been researched extensively. A basal approach would also most likely be more successful than learning to read strictly by a whole language or trade books. Newer basal series are incorporating the use of leveled readers (short books on a given topic) to differentiate the instruction within the classroom. These series have computer components, as well as listening tapes, fluency practice, and skills pages to offer more flexibility in meeting each student's needs. In addition, they offer spelling and language instruction related to the skills taught in each unit.

The Scott-Foresman reading program entitled Reading Street is a good example of this type of basal program. This program also has the added bonus of drawing many of its reading selections from nonfiction sources. At the primary level 50% of the readings are nonfiction and at the upper elementary this number increases to 60%. This approach would benefit the VCFS student by exposing them to stories about real life situations and science and social studies topics. These selections can give a foundation for understanding the curriculum taught in these content areas. This basal series also has a direct instruction component for struggling readers and a sound recognition computer program to assist with fluency. Reading using a computer screen has advantages for students with VCFS who may visually benefit from changes in the size of the font.

Giving students with VCFS multiple opportunities to practice skills in a small group or one-to-one setting works well regardless of what reading program is adopted. It also helps for these children to read books multiple times in order to build a sight vocabulary. Children with VCFS will typically require additional practice to commit a skill to memory, so patience and extended time for assignments is needed. In the lower elementary grades, where the focus is on decoding, children with VCFS can function pretty well. In later years, where comprehension skills are needed, the gap between the student with VCFS and his or her peers widens. Laying a foundation for understanding language can be accomplished both in the classroom and with speech and language therapy. Guided reading practice with fill-in-the-blank exercises is just one example of an approach that would actively involve the learner. The technique of discussion of a story in the large group circle would not be as beneficial for children with VCFS because of their difficulty with auditory processing skills. In addition, they may not fully understand the language of the discussion or be able to follow a quickly paced conversation. Brain imaging studies (see Chapter 3) also indicated a problem with storing a thought mentally and then applying that thought to another situation. Thus, if the teacher asks students to think about the characters in the story and then predict how these characters would react in a different situation, a child with VCFS would have trouble responding. A better approach would be to list attributes of the character, separately discuss the new situation, and then refer to the written list to predict how the character would react. This would break down the task and free up memory to apply toward solving the problem.

Retelling stories can be much more difficult than simply reading the words. This is an area of weakness for the VCFS population. Using a template with specific questions can help a child remember pertinent story facts. Word banks, tape recorders, and visual clues can also help them recall the important aspects of a story. Educators should keep in mind the difficulty with storing and retrieving large amounts of information and develop strategies of recording smaller chunks of needed information. Visual templates, like story maps, should be used to help the student record pertinent information. As the child matures, there are additional techniques that can be used to enhance comprehension (see Comprehension section in Chapter 11).

Using trade books in conjunction with more structured reading instruction can help instill a joy in reading and can certainly be incorporated into a reading program. In addition, reading other short trade books like *The Berenstain Bears and the Messy Room* by Stan and Jan Berenstain can also serve a dual purpose of teaching daily living skills. These books, along with additional activities, are available at http://www.berenstainbears.com. Reading aloud to an adult can be very motivating to students with VCFS. Decoding words is an area of strength and working on fluency on a regular basis will help with reading comprehension skills.

## WRITTEN LANGUAGE, SPELLING, AND ORAL COMMUNICATION

Creative writing, grammar, and spelling are relatively strong for the typical child with VCFS. Rote practice with conventions, memorizing spelling lists, and opportunities to create stories come more easily than other academic tasks. Using a sensory approach to spelling can facilitate memorizing words. Students can trace words on sandpaper, in sand, or on other surfaces to stimulate the tactile senses. Fine motor coordination may be difficult so the process of actually forming the letters on paper can complicate the writing process. As soon as feasible, learning to use a computer to keyboard is helpful. In the primary grades, however, an adult can act as a scribe to help put on paper the child's creative ideas. Some teachers also use the Rebecca Sitton Spelling Program to help young students master core words. Focusing on a core number of commonly used words also simplifies the spelling task.

Expressive and receptive language skills usually are areas that need remediation by speech and language professionals. Children with VCFS have deficits in understanding the meaning of space and time words such as between, behind, and before. They may not understand idioms (such as *for the birds* or *see eye to eye*) and are very concrete in their thinking. They also have trouble retelling events that happened in school and adding detail to their writings or conversations. Word banks, story outlines, templates, and pictures for clues are all possible accommodations. Educators should also be in close contact with parents and provide written communication because children with VCFS often cannot provide this home-school connection on their own.

## COMPUTERS

Computer skills should be taught as early as feasible. Many children with VCFS do quite well with keyboarding and they find that creative writing is much more enjoyable done on a computer. They can free their minds to focus on their compositions rather than on struggling with the fine motor writing task. With continued practice, many are quite adept at both keyboarding and computer use. Computers also work well to reinforce basic skills. Programs that offer drill and practice with math facts are effective, as are reading comprehension programs.

## MATHEMATICS

Mathematics is a universal area of weakness with velo-cardio-facial syndrome. Most educators typically view math as a hierarchical subject. That is, early skills must be established before further skills can be mastered (C. Mercer, Jordan & Miller, 1994).

According to Piaget (1959), C. Mercer et al. (1994), and C. Mercer and A. Mercer (1997), basic skill acquisition should focus on the following areas:

1. Classification—the ability to sort and classify according to color, shape, size, or use

2. Number conservation—the ability to understand the amounts remain the same when appearances change (the amount of cereal in a box completely poured into a bowl remains the same)

3. One-to-one correspondence—the ability to understand that one object in a set is the same number as one object in another set (e.g., seven oranges represents the same quantity as seven apples)

4. Ordering—the ability to arrange items based on a particular property (such as length or quantity)

Recent research in teaching mathematics to students with mathematical disabilities has called for a shift from the typical drill and practice approach to one that emphasizes the development of number sense (Gersten & Chard, 1999). Number sense refers to a child's understanding of what numbers mean, an ability to do mental calculations, and the ability to look at the world and make accurate comparisons. Children with good number sense can move with ease from the real world of quantities to the mathematical world of numbers and expressions. They can represent the same number in multiple ways, can recognize number patterns, have a good sense of number magnitude, can estimate, and can see gross numerical errors. They have many strategies for solving problems and can invent their own procedures for doing math operations (Case, 1998). Children with VCFS will have difficulty inventing their own strategies, but can be taught these techniques using direct instruction. An example of a strategy is the use of "min strategy" for addition. Children recognize that when adding $7 + 2$ it is easier to begin with the larger number 7 and then add 2, rather than the other way around $(2 + 7)$. Another strategy for addition of several digits involves grouping the numbers by sums that equal ten. $3 + 8 + 7 + 2 + 7 = ?$ can easily be solved by grouping $(7 + 3) + (2 + 8)$ and then adding the remaining 7, rather than adding the numbers as they appear in the problem. Children who do not acquire number sense before kindergarten need formal instruction to do so (Bruer, 1997).

The previous chapter (Chapter 8) discussed several readiness skills, including number sense, that are necessary before a child can advance to more complicated math operations. Students should be assessed as to whether these concepts have been mastered, and if not, remediation is necessary. Any of the interventions previously detailed (Number Worlds, On Cloud Nine, Singapore Math) would be appropriate to continue. Students with VCFS will need multiple opportunities for hands-on practice with these concepts. Discovery math programs do not work effectively with this population. Children with VCFS have great difficulty seeing the big picture or intuitively grasping math concepts. Direct instruction, where relationships are demonstrated and skills are taught with concrete examples, works better. They also need a step-by-step approach where one skill builds on the next, along with a lot of repetition. Spiraling curriculums that introduce many skills with limited practice opportunities are less effective.

Early special education research in the 1980s by Goldman, Pelligrino and Mertz (1988) and Goldman (1989) looked at automaticity of basic facts and the effect on achievement. It was concluded that reaching automaticity, a level of proficiency where skill execution is rapid or automatic with little or no conscious monitoring, is correlated with math competence. Special education teachers were encouraged to focus remediation efforts on extended practice on memorizing math facts. While more current research suggests additional remedial strategies are necessary, automaticity is still an important aspect in gaining math mastery.

Mastering basic facts and rote calculations are usually strengths for students with VCFS. Although initially committing facts to memory will be time intensive, it is worth the effort. A good foundation in basic facts will offer opportunities for the child with VCFS to have some success with more complex math tasks. Automatic recall will also allow the child with VCFS to free more brain space to tackle more difficult problem solving. As discussed earlier in the book, imaging studies involving children with VCFS showed inefficiencies in processing math operations (Eliez, 2001). Working to "rewire" the brain to make factual recall more efficient will lessen the attentional demand and allow the freed resources to be allocated to other tasks or higher-order thinking functions. Computer games, music CDs, flash cards, and drill all work to solidify recall of basic facts.

The Kumon Institute of Education of Japan offers an after-school program in math and reading throughout many cities in the United States and abroad. The program is intended to supplement the skills taught in school through a method of repeated drill and practice. The program, written by a man whose son had Down syndrome, originated in Japan. The father, determined to find a technique that worked to teach his child, developed an incremental system to mastering math skills. He broke each task down to small steps and through daily practice the child masters more and more difficult calculations. The math program is primarily computation based and goes from elementary skills through calculus. Students have short daily assignments to do on skills and they work for speed and mastery. It is individualized and students repeat pages until they can do the work quickly and correctly. Since the children work at their own pace, they can spend as much time as they need to memorize the facts. The repeated, daily practice is a method that is most likely to succeed. This program has been successfully used with students with VCFS to help solidify basic facts. Information about the Kumon program is available at http://www.kumon.com.

In summary, effective teaching of math in the school setting will need to combine direct instruction (teacher initiated tasks, modeling) with strategy instruction (study skills, memorization techniques, different ways to solve problems, new methods to approach learning). The approach to instruction should include:

- Repetition and practice (automatizing math facts, daily practice, sequenced review)

- Sequencing and task analysis (break larger problems into steps, provide prompts, synthesize the parts into a whole)

- Instruction in the linguistic components of math

- One-on-one or small group discussions of concepts (structured questioning where the instructor can build instruction in incremental steps and can recheck for understanding)

- Incremental task difficulty (teacher should sequence problems from easy to difficult)

- Teacher-modeled problem solving

- Use of computer assisted learning

- Reminders to use strategies

- Assistance generalizing problems to other situations

Math learning sessions should also include the following:

- Oral practice with math facts
- Practice with visualizing problems
- Remedial instruction in prerequisite skills if necessary
- Verbalizing of math concepts by child
- Estimation and number sense practice
- Practice counting forwards and backwards beginning with various numbers (by 2s, 3s, etc.)
- Practice with number fact patterns (ex. 5 + 5 = 10, then 5 + 6 + 5 = 10 + 6 or 16)

Finally, many math skills are best acquired using real world applications. For example, the concept of money could be taught using play coins at a classroom store. The actual tactile experience of handling the coins in a real situation would prove more meaningful. The approach to telling time should involve actual clocks that can be manipulated and perhaps situated at the child's desk. Keep in mind that life skill applications are an extremely important aspect of these children's curriculum. Any opportunity to make connections between school tasks and life situations would be beneficial.

## CONTENT AREAS—SOCIAL STUDIES AND SCIENCE

Science and social studies in the primary grades usually focus on building a foundation to understand the world around us. Concrete concepts with real life examples would help children with VCFS make connections to their lives. Preferential seating during any class discussions would help with focusing attention. Teachers must also keep in mind, however, that children with VCFS will gain little from oral discussions without practicing the skills. They must be given some type of active learning activity to begin to process the information. Talking about insects or reading from a book will be ineffective compared to making insect models or catching and observing a real specimen. Any concept that needs to be learned should be clearly communicated to the students, to the parents, and to the special education teacher. For example, if the children are supposed to understand after the lesson that insects have three body parts and six legs, this needs to be written out. This concept then can be discussed and reinforced one-on-one at speech therapy and at home. In addition, new vocabulary for the lesson should be pretaught, if possible. Mastery of unfamiliar words, in advance, will help the student with VCFS participate more meaningfully in discussions. Again, remember the key to learning is repetition, modeling, and multiple practice opportunities.

# SOCIAL SKILLS/LIFE SKILLS

Studies focusing on children and adults with VCFS show many deficits in the areas of social skills development and the mastering of life skills. Primary classrooms usually include some instruction in these areas, but children with VCFS need a more intensive approach. They do not learn by simply observing and often do not make the connection between their actions and consequences that follow. Many parents describe their children as lacking common sense. Adults wrongly assume that they should know better or can figure things out on their own. In fact, many children with VCFS must be taught these skills directly.

Interventions that are successful for teaching social interaction skills include social stories, social scripts, the Situation Options Consequences Choices Strategies Simulation (SOCCSS), direct instruction, role playing, and supervised play groups.

## Social Stories

In 1991, Carol Gray designed the technique of social stories while working with a child with autism. She observed that the child was confused and disoriented by a game his class was learning during gym. She wrote a story describing the rules to the game and the responses the other children had to playing. The autistic child practiced reading the story several times for a week. The following week, when the child returned to gym class he understood the game, actively participated, and enjoyed the activity. Thus, the concept of writing social stories was born.

From that initial activity guidelines were developed for writing these stories that would help make them effective and practical to use. The social story is specific to an individual and to circumstances. It describes a social situation and includes directive statements that model appropriate behaviors for the setting. *The Original Social Stories Book* contains stories about a variety of social situations including stories about home (such as helping around the house, bedtime, babysitters, cooking, free time), school (teachers, academics, recess, lunch), and the community (getting around, community helpers, shopping, recreation). It also includes a template for writing original social stories in response to individual student needs. These needs can be identified by observing situations that are difficult for the student, by social skills assessments, and by noting students' responses to questions that indicate he or she is misreading the situation. The stories describe the situation, emphasize the social skills needed, identify appropriate interactions, teach routines, and help teach academic material in a realistic, social backdrop.

# BEHAVIOR ISSUES, HEALTH CONCERNS, AND ADDITIONAL PROGRAMS TO ADDRESS SELF-REGULATION

Behavior issues associated with VCFS can be an obstacle to learning and can undermine efforts to succeed in school. Frustration, poor attention skills, lower cognitive ability, learned helplessness, delayed motor skills, and poor problem-solving skills are just some of the contributing factors to school difficulties. In addition, chronic health difficulties translate into missed instruction due to absences and doctor appointments. Moreover, when the student is able to attend school, he or she may have chronic ear infections, lethargy, poor muscle tone, leg pains, and various other health-related problems. All of these issues may affect school performance and classroom behavior.

School personnel can assist the child and family by instituting programs within the school to help. One program, described earlier, involves the How Does Your Engine Run program for sensory regulation (see Chapter 9). Another program designed to improve cognitive integration, attention, and behavior is called Bal-A-Vis-X: Rhythmic, Balance/Auditory/Vision Exercises for Brain and Brain-Body Integration by Bill Hubert. The program uses exercises with rhythm, sound, and balls to improve listening skills, visual difficulties (ocular motility or tracking), binocularity or teaming, visual form perception (discrimination of details), and attention. The exercises are similar to juggling and are done alone, with partners, or in teams of several students. As the activities increase in complexity, students become more able to focus visually and auditorily. Some schools train the gym teacher to teach these exercises during physical education and other districts rely on the occupational or physical therapist.

Another program closely related to the Bal-A-Vis-X is Brain Gym, written by Paul Dennison. The premise of this program is that kinesiology can be applied to the process of cognitive development and learning. The philosophy of Brain Gym suggests that certain physical movements can restore proper energy flow from brain to muscle and from muscle to brain. Movements can facilitate communication among and integration of the various hemispheres of the brain and in turn improve academic skills, behavior, and attention. Specific movements target particular skills. For example, before doing math, students would do the exercises designed to improve the ability to compute. Information about this program including research studies regarding its effectiveness can be obtained at http://www.braingym.org.

## CASE VIGNETTES

Even with the best intentions, programs for children with VCFS can be complicated to design. The following cases illustrate two scenarios.

## Case 1

Matt was a 6-year-old boy with VCFS who lived with his parents on the east coast of the United States. He had a congenital heart defect (truncus arteriosus), hypotonia, gastroesophageal reflux disease, a compromised immune system, and a history of oral feeding intolerance. He also had a history of chronic ear infections, had been identified as developmentally delayed, and had difficulty with attention. He had a FSIQ of 78, PIQ 73, and VIQ of 83. Kindergarten teachers reported that Matt had difficulty with self-help, fine motor skills, and staying on task. His language skills were delayed and he was difficult to understand. He was placed in a regular half-day kindergarten because the special education pull-out kindergarten had children who seemed more severely cognitively impaired. His classroom had 21 children and no aide. Matt received 30 minutes of speech therapy a week, OT 30 minutes per week, and behavioral counseling 1 hour per week. Academically he was a year behind the peers in his class.

At the end of the kindergarten year, an independent evaluator recommended that Matt attend a full-day kindergarten the next year rather than enter first grade. The decision, however, was made to have Matt move on to first grade with his same-age peers. His assistance from the special education staff was increased to 2 hours per day (an hour each for math and language). He also continued with speech and language therapy (30 minutes per week) and OT therapy (15 minutes per week). At the end of first grade, the teachers reported gains academically, but that Matt continued to struggle with math, reading comprehension, on-task behavior, and his ability to follow a chain of directions. He needed one-on-one attention to complete assignments and his communication skills were lacking. Many accommodations were written into the educational plan including, but not limited to: giving Matt additional help after presentations, reducing writing demands, reducing visual clutter on assignments, modifying expectation for work, use of an assignment notebook, preferential seating, etc. The issue of repeating a grade was discussed. Matt's parents were concerned about his progress and looked into private school settings with smaller class sizes and additional services. The parents felt the school was making a good effort meeting Matt's needs, but because of limited resources he was not really getting the assistance that he needed throughout much of the day.

## Case 2

Cory was a second-grade student with VCFS from a southern U.S. school district. He had been receiving special education services since preschool. He had a heart murmur, velopharyngeal incompetence, enamel hypoplasia, short stature, motor deficit, severe articulation delay, and hyperkeratosis. He exhibited moderate delays in cognition, expressive language, gross and fine motor skills, and self-care skills.

Cory's first-grade year went relatively well. He struggled in math and written language, but for the most part he was making progress and keeping up with his classmates. By the first quarter of second grade, however, he was receiving failing grades for math, reading, and social studies. Written communication between home and school revealed a rather rigid approach to learning by the school. Cory's mother reported that he was overwhelmed with the amount of homework (at least three subjects a night) and he often broke down crying. She was concerned with the school's punitive approach for late work and misplaced papers. The school responded that they required the same work from their special education students as from the regular students, and if the homework wasn't done, Cory would face the consequences at school. None of Cory's papers had positive comments written on them; most just contained check marks and letters grades (which were mostly Fs). Cory was also reprimanded for not keeping his papers organized and filed properly. He began to resist going to school.

Although Cory was making progress the previous year, the pace of instruction and the expectations of the staff were clearly making school a negative experience for a very young student. After the parents enlisted the help of an educational consultant versed in VCFS, the staff better understood the challenges Cory faced and revised their approach to working with him. They increased the amount of help he received at school and made adjustments to his workload. At last report, he was making progress and going to school willingly.

## REFERENCES

Adams, G. L., & Engelmann, S. (1996). *Research on direct instruction: 25 years beyond DISTAR*. Seattle, WA: Educational Achievement Systems.

Bruer, J. T. (1997). Education and the brain: A bridge too far. *Educational Researcher, 26*(8), 4–16.

Case, R. (1998, April). *A psychological model of number sense and its development*. Paper presented at the annual meeting of the American Educational Research Association, San Diego, CA.

Dennison, P., & Dennison, G. (1994). *Brain gym*. Ventura, CA: Edu-Kinesthetics.

Eliez, S., Blasey, C. M., Menon, V., White, C. D., Schmitt, J. E., & Reiss, A. L. (2001). Functional brain imaging study of mathematical reasoning abilities in velocardiofacial syndrome (del. 22q11.2). *Genetics in Medicine, 3*(1), 49–55.

Forness, S. R., Kavale, K. A., Blum, I. M., & Lloyd, J. W. (1997). Mega-analysis of meta-analyses: What works in special education. *Teaching Exceptional Children, 29*(6), 4–9.

Gersten, R., & Chard, D. (1999). Number sense: Rethinking arithmetic instruction for students with mathematical disabilities. *The Journal of Special Education, 44*, 18–28.

Goldman, S. R., Pellegrino, J. W., & Mertz, D. L. (1988). Extended practice of basic addition facts: Strategy changes in learning-disabled students. *Cognition and Instruction, 5*(3), 225–265.

Goldman, S. R. (1989). Strategy instruction in mathematics. *Learning Disability Quartery, 12*(1), 43–55.

Gray, C. (1993). *The original social story book*. Arlington, TX: Future Horizons.

Harvey, S., & Goudvis, A. (2000) *Strategies that work, teaching comprehension to enhance understanding*. Portland, ME: Stenhouse.

Hubert, B. (2001). *Bal-A-Vis-X, Rhythmic, balance/auditory/vision exercises for brain and brain-body integration*. Wichita, KS: Bal-A-Vis-X.

Kaminski, R., & Good, R. (1996). *Phoneme segmentation fluency (Dynamic Indicators of Basic Early Literacy Skills [DIBELS])*. Austin, TX: Pro-Ed.

Piaget, J. (1959). *The language and thought of the child*. London: Routledge.

Mercer, C., Jordan, L., & Miller, S. (1994). Implications of constructivism for teaching math to students with moderate to mild disabilities. *The Journal of Special Education, 28*(3), 290–306.

Mercer, C., & Mercer, A. (1997). *Teaching students with learning problems*. Englewood Cliffs, NJ: Prentice Hall.

National Reading Panel (2000). Teaching children to read: An evidenced-based assessment of the scientific research literature on reading and its implication for reading instruction: Reports of the subgroups: Washington DC: National Institute of Child Health and Development.

Stanovich, K. E. (2000). *Progress in understanding reading: Scientific foundations and new frontiers*. New York, NY: Guilford Press.

Tarver, S. (1999). Focusing on direct instruction. *Current Practice Alerts, Division for Learning Disabilities and Division for Research, 2*(2).

Torgensen, J., & Bryant, B. (1994). Test of Phonological Awareness. Austin, TX: Pro-Ed.

Vaughn, S., & Linan-Thompson, S. (2004). Research-based methods of reading instruction. Alexandria, VA: Association for Supervision and Curriculum Development.

Wagner, R., Torgensen, J., & Rashotte, C. (1999). *Comprehensive Test of Phonological Processing*. Austin, TX: Pro-Ed.

Williams, M., & Shellenberger, S. (1996). *How does your engine run? A leader's guide to the alert program for self-regulation*. Albuquerque, NM: Therapy Works.

Yopp, H. (1995) Yopp-Singer Test of Phoneme Segmentation, *Reading Teacher, 49*(1), 20–29.

# BIBLIOGRAPHY/SUGGESTED READINGS

Au, K., Carroll, & Scheu, J. (1997). *Balanced literacy instruction: A teacher's resource book*. Norwood, MA: Christopher-Gordon Publishers.

Beaver, J. (2001). *Developmental reading assessment: K–3 teacher resource guide*. Parsippany, NJ: Celebration Press.

Fountas, I. C., & Pinnell, G. S. (1996). *Guided reading, Good first teaching for all children*. Portsmouth, NH: Heinemann.

Galvin, M. (1995). *Otto learns about his medicine: A story about medication for children with ADHD*. Washington, DC, Magination Press.

Hiebert, J. (1997). *Making sense: Teaching and learning mathematics with understanding*. Portsmouth, NH, Heinemann.

Miller, D. (2002). *Reading with meaning: Teaching comprehension in the primary grades*. Portland, ME: Stenhouse.

Mills, J. (1992). *Little tree. A story for children with serious medical problems*. Washington, DC: Magination Press.

Pinnell, G. S., & Scharer, P.L. (2003). *Teaching for comprehension in reading*. New York: Scholastic.

Prestine, J. S., & Kylberg, V. (1993). *Sometimes I feel awful*. Carthage, IL: Fearon Teacher Aids.

Salinger, T. S. (1993). *Models of literacy instruction*. New York Toronto, Merrill; Maxwell Macmillan Canada; Maxwell Macmillan International.

Tomlinson, C. A., & Eidson, C. C. (2003). *Differentiation in practice, A resource guide for differentiating curriculum, Grades K–5*. Alexandria, VA: Association for Supervision and Curriculum Development.

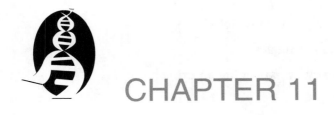

# CHAPTER 11

# Gaining Expertise

## *Upper Elementary Grades Three through Five (Ages 8–11)*

As elementary school continues, students are asked to assume more responsibility for independent work, use higher level thinking skills, and master more comprehensive curriculum. The shift from rote memorization tasks to those requiring abstract reasoning and critical thinking can be quite daunting for a child with VCFS. Many children find that school becomes much more difficult and parents struggle with how to effectively help their child at home. Both educators and parents need to realize that the primary learning deficits associated with this syndrome (i.e., working memory, math reasoning, reading comprehension, etc.) often do not manifest themselves until this time. Therefore, it is imperative that students are carefully screened for increasing school difficulties.

Some indicators of problems are:

- Trouble understanding or following verbal directions in class

- Late or missing assignments

- Unfinished work

- Frequent uncertainty of how to proceed with an assignment

- Work attempted, but done incorrectly

- Quietness in class—doesn't ask or answer questions often

- Looking to others to help or guide them

■ Math reasoning or story problem deficits

■ Reading comprehension struggles

■ Difficulty retelling a story or explaining an event

■ Social/behavior problems

Teachers of older children can continue to use the same classroom environment suggestions, sensory techniques, and academic strategies suggested earlier for younger children. There may be some modifications necessary, but in general the suggestions are applicable to this age level also.

The major shift at this age is the expectation by teachers that students can follow multiple oral directions, work efficiently and independently, and have acquired the prerequisite skills to do more advanced work.

As discussed earlier, brain abnormalities in VCFS subjects hinder their ability to process ideas efficiently. In addition, when presented with a multiple-step problem to solve, VCFS subjects needed to recruit considerably more brainpower than normal subjects. They also needed to use different parts of their brains to process this information. When one translates these findings to a classroom setting, it can explain some of the trouble students at this age demonstrate with following multistep directions and complex discussions. Simply put, the pace of instruction is too quick for a child with VCFS to keep up. This does *not* mean that the content is too difficult. What it does mean, however, is that accommodations must be made in order for children with VCFS to benefit from the instruction.

## ACCOMMODATIONS FOR WORKING MEMORY DEFICITS

Many classroom accommodations are possible to allow the child with VCFS to participate in the regular academic curriculum. The most important is the concept of slowed reteaching in a one-on-one or small group setting. This can be accomplished in a resource model special education program or through an inclusion model with a special educator or aide available to assist in the regular classroom. The child must be able to have the instruction broken down to manageable parts that he or she can process and store in memory. In a large group setting, children with VCFS will miss a large bulk of the presentation. They may look like they are paying attention, but when questioned they often will not remember or understand what was taught. They also will miss a good deal of information presented by video, during discussions, or covered by the teacher instructing the large class. Direct instruction, with a simplified step-by-step model, will help make the content more meaningful. In addition, it will allow the child to process the information at a speed he or she can tolerate. It will also allow the adult to check frequently for understanding and then adjust the instruction accordingly. Memory cues such as lists, word banks, and visual step-by-step charts also help make the learning less frustrating.

Children with VCFS also learn best by *doing* rather than observing others or listening to class discussions. They *must* be actively involved in the activity in order for them to grasp the content. Active learning also helps them sustain attention and be accountable for their work. Making the curriculum meaningful is also very helpful. For example, some elementary schools operate a school store where students can purchase school supplies. Working in this type of setting to learn how to make change or figure the cost of a purchase would be a beneficial approach. Educators should keep in mind that most children with VCFS will need assistance with life skills. Any opportunity to relate the curriculum to real life experiences will be particularly helpful preparing these students for life on their own.

Multiple repetitions are necessary to encode new information into memory. Since many children with VCFS must use different parts of their brains than normal to do learning tasks, they are not efficient learners. This doesn't mean that they can't master a skill, but rather that it will take more time and effort. It will also take many repetitions to "rewire" the brain to be able to retrieve this information and use it later. Drill and practice are needed to make these new connections. It is also necessary to keep building on and reusing these skills so they are not lost. Care should be taken not to overload the student with too much new information at once. Shorter study periods over several days are preferable to one long study time. Building in review as a new concept is introduced is also encouraged to keep learned skills fresh and accessible.

Write down all directions for the student and provide notes and study guides. Children with VCFS need information written down so adults helping them understand the assignments and so they can remind themselves what they are to do. Do not expect these students to take notes or to remember oral directions. Typically, they are unable to do this even given their best effort. In addition, as students move through fifth grade they are often expected to remember content for tests in science and social studies. Children with VCFS will need the curriculum they are required to master in *written form*. It would be best to also condense the content they have to memorize to the most important information. Try not to make memorizing information a large part of their grade and recognize the huge amount of effort it takes for a student with VCFS to successfully memorize content.

Other techniques to help with a working memory deficit include:

- Using a tape recorder while reading to remember previous parts of a book.

- Allowing word banks on tests to help with recall.

- Providing guided reading sheets to help with comprehension of material.

- Providing a template for multistep problems so a child can record any answers needed to finish solving the problem. This way a child doesn't have to keep these answers in working memory.

- Teaching a system of recording assignments—use a classroom chart along with an assignment notebook so students can copy down what they need to do. Teachers should then check the child's book for accuracy.

- Keeping a schedule on the child's desk of all transitions so the child can refer to this and not rely on remembering the daily activities.

- See Appendix A for more suggestions.

### Cognitive Remediation Therapy

Several recent studies are showing improvement of cognitive deficits through the use of cognitive remediation therapies. Although in the past, working memory was thought to be constant, new investigations are suggesting that working memory can be improved by training (Olesen, Westerberg, & Klingberg, 2004; C. Stevenson, Whitmont, Bornholt, Livesey, & R. Stevenson, 2002). Additional studies involving patients with schizophrenia have also shown promising results in improved cognitive function after several weeks of cognitive therapy (Wykes et al., 2002). Cognitive remediation therapy has not been studied with the VCFS population or extensively with young children, but there are studies that support rehearsal-based training for improved short-term memory in children with Down syndrome (Broadley & MacDonald, 1993; Broadley, MacDonald, & Buckley, 1999). There have also been positive results seen using computerized training of working memory with children with ADHD (Klingberg et. al., 2005). Cognitive remediation has also been examined with pediatric cancer patients who have learning problems after receiving radiation and chemotherapies. The preliminary result of these studies is also promising (Copeland & Butler, 2002). This area needs more study, but there are programs currently available that may offer some assistance.

Cognitive remediation focuses on three key areas:

- Cognitive flexibility—the ability to switch from one task to another. Example: The ability to correctly delete odd and then even numbers from a list.

- Working memory—thinking about one task while doing another. Example: The ability to remember a sequence of colored disks and then line them up in a different order.

- Planning ahead. Example: The ability to plan ahead when moving a set of tokens to a new position following a set of rules.

One program available for schools to address these skill areas is the Structure of Intellect System. The program is marketed under the Bridges trade name and is also known as SOI (http://www.soisystems.com or http://www.bridges learning.com). It is based on the work of J. P. Guilford and has been used in schools for over 35 years. This system attempts to increase the capacity to learn by assessing 27 different thinking abilities. It then offers specific activities to remediate deficiencies. In addition to remedial programs for reading and math, the SOI system has a Memory Matrix computer program. The goal of this program is to help develop memory for visual relations, details, complex relations, whole words, and verbal comprehension. Another program area strengthens memory abilities by improving skills like remembering objects, words, sets of numbers backward and forwards, words in sentences, and classifying word lists into categories. The primary program components are appropriate for ages 7 and up, but there are preschool and home activities as well. There are some studies that support the efficacy of this program (http://www.upsidedownschoolroom.com/soi-research.shtml), but more studies will be needed to see if it is effective with the VCFS population.

In addition to cognitive remediation therapy, mnemonics can also be used to enhance memory retrieval. The next chapter (Chapter 12) on middle school interventions discusses the use of mnemonics more in depth. However, memory techniques are helpful as learning strategies at this age, also.

## ORGANIZATION AND STUDY SKILLS

Many of the major skills taught in upper elementary school center on readiness for attending a middle or junior high school. There, students often move from teacher to teacher and must have a system for keeping track of their assignments and supplies. For students with working memory impairments and with executive planning struggles this aspect of school is particularly troublesome. They just can't seem to make it all work. Their desks are disorganized, they forget needed materials at school, and they are unclear on what is due the next day. Teachers who penalize for late work add to the frustration level, and by the time these students get to middle school they feel like failures. Many give up trying because the tasks just seem insurmountable. Flexibility is the key to making school a positive experience for a child with VCFS. Although responsibility for homework may be a realistic goal for the typically developing fifth grader, it is likely an unrealistic expectation for a student with VCFS. Students *should* be held accountable for assignments, but teachers may need to give these students extra assistance to accomplish this. Students should not be scolded for forgetting materials or assignments, but rather given a written reminder of what is due. If directions were misinterpreted, students should be given an opportunity to redo or correct the assignment. Remember, the goal is to foster a love for learning and a positive sense of self and to help a child with VCFS continue to strive to succeed. Teachers should have high expectations. However, they must also recognize and reward effort—especially in children who are struggling with so many deficits.

There are several ways to assist a disorganized student with managing papers and assignments. First, it is imperative that he or she has an assignment notebook to record assignments that are due. Fourth and fifth graders can be taught how to fill these books out and many students become quite proficient in this task. There is also an erasable homework chart the teacher can post in the classroom that looks like an assignment notebook page. A chart called the Homework Master is available from the Success by Design Company. Teachers (or classroom student helpers) can record the daily assignments and the due dates for the class to copy. It is also helpful if teachers go over the chart orally with prompts to take out needed supplies for individual assignments. *Children with VCFS will need the additional step of having the teacher check over their assignment book and make sure they have the needed materials gathered to take home.* Many assignment books also have a spot for parents to initial that they have checked over the assignments due. Parents can also help by making sure the child places all the needed work in the backpack for school the next day. This home-school connection is imperative and will eliminate many unnecessary difficulties over homework completion.

Another technique that is successful in helping students keep track of their papers is the use of the accordion folder. This folder replaces a Trapper Keeper or loose folders for different subjects. One large folder is used that has several tabs or compartments. Each compartment would correspond to a different subject (reading, language, spelling, science, etc.). Students file all papers in the appropriate slot. One slot is also reserved for take-home notices. Accordion folders should be cleaned out after each week and graded papers can be stored at home if needed for a future test or tossed. Students take accordion folders with them as they change classes through the day. This system seems to eliminate many lost papers and messy desks. The folders are readily available at office supply or discount stores.

In addition, students need a system both at home and at school for organizing their supplies. Children with VCFS should be taught a routine for keeping their areas free of clutter. I have noticed that students who take a couple extra seconds to file their papers as soon as they move on to another subject are much better organized. This method of constant organizing works much better than the alternative of carelessly dealing with papers and then doing a cleaning all at one time. Having a definite place for all supplies and papers helps this process, too. Students should have a study area at home, just as they do at school, where they do their homework and store their papers. Children with VCFS also must learn to put their homework into their backpacks as soon as they complete it. Leaving the job of collecting due assignments for the morning before school is a recipe for disaster. Students anxious about being late or missing the bus or simply distracted will likely leave the completed assignment on their desk at home!

Finally, children with VCFS will need help with organizing their time as well as their supplies. Helping families set a routine for homework helps and so does having a monthly calendar to post appointments, sports commitments, family activities, etc. Fifth graders also will need help budgeting their time in order to complete long-term assignments such as book reports or science fair projects. Parents and teachers will need to actively break these long-term due dates to shorter time periods. Small goals, such as reading five pages a night, become much more workable. Do not assume children with VCFS will be able to figure this out alone. They will likely need adult intervention with this skill, perhaps into adulthood. Planning, problem solving, and executive functioning are usually impaired in this population, so accommodations to address this will be needed.

## HOMEWORK AND REMEDIATION

Children with VCFS will need to spend considerable time outside of school working on learning skills. The time spent in additional academic study will be well worth the investment. In many cases, it will mean the difference of a chance to be enrolled in a post-secondary training program and/or gainfully employed as an adult. Establishing good study habits in upper elementary school helps the child prepare for the demands of middle and high school. It also gives additional drill and practice opportunities and cements basic skills.

Students who have difficulty settling down to do homework or who are in need of remediation can be helped with a set homework time every day Monday through Thursday. This can be from 30 minutes to 1 hour. Children who do not have a school assignment to complete can use this time to do other academic related activities. Some suggestions might be practicing math facts, reading a book, playing an educational computer game, or writing in a diary. Most children with VCFS will need this extra academic practice to keep their skills sharp. Parents can supervise this study time or might consider hiring a tutor to work with their child.

Many parents find that hiring a tutor to help their child is worth the additional cost. Often children will more readily cooperate with a tutor and tend to whine and complain more to a parent. Parents also can become frustrated working with a child who is experiencing learning difficulties. Educating this type of learner takes patience, humor, and experience. Many parents have a difficult time when their child cannot master material as quickly as other children. This can lead to a damaging relationship and hurt feelings. Having a third party work with the child with VCFS will allow the parent to step back from this situation and assume the role as parent, not teacher. Schools can also assist by offering after-school homework clubs or perhaps enlisting the help of a community mentor to assist the child with homework completion.

Finding a tutor is usually fairly easy. Parents can call their child's school for a list of names. Another possibility is to contact a local college or university to see if it has a job posting area. Often, students in the fields of education or special education will be very willing to work one-on-one with a special needs child. This experience will be a valuable addition to a student's resume and will provide some needed cash as well. Other parents may also know of adults in the community who offer tutoring services.

Another avenue to explore is to enroll the child with VCFS in an after-school academic program. One suggestion mentioned earlier is the Kumon Math and Reading Program. Several VCFS families have had success with this particular program. The math philosophy was discussed in Chapter 10 and can easily be continued throughout elementary and middle school. The Kumon reading program consists of vocabulary, comprehension, and short answer written responses. It has a global emphasis and the selection of literature is rich with an international flavor. The format of the pages is excellent for a child with VCFS. Each page is uncluttered with a small selection to read. The reading program also moves to harder concepts in small, linear steps—one skill building upon the next. The Kumon program allows each child, regardless of age, to progress at a comfortable speed. Both special needs and gifted students have benefited from the Kumon approach and all ranges of abilities enroll in the centers.

Another program that has been used by students with VCFS is the Fast ForWord intervention for struggling readers. This program developed by Scientific Learning, http://www.scilearn.com, is a computer-based program designed to improve memory, attention, processing, and sequencing skills through computerized games. Students develop critical reading skills including phonemic awareness, fluency, vocabulary, comprehension, decoding, and syntax. The program is completed in an intensive 8- to 12-week period with the help of an independent speech and language professional or through the school system. Privately, the program is expensive. However, the company has conducted several scientific studies that give positive results.

## ACADEMICS IN UPPER ELEMENTARY SCHOOL

### Reading

Students in upper elementary school are solidifying basic skills and moving from needing assistance with reading to being independent learners. Reading emphasis shifts from decoding and oral fluency to understanding concepts like cause and effect, inferences, and story elements. The expectations are higher and detailed, and complete answers to comprehension questions require careful reading and interpretations. Students are taught the structure of plots, character analysis, and setting characteristics. By age 10, most children can read easier novels independently for enjoyment. Many literature assignments ask students to summarize plots, to give opinions as to the author's purpose for writing the selection, and to relate the reading to historical events. Reading also becomes a primary source of gathering information in the content areas of social studies and science.

Children with VCFS will likely need a more intensive reading program in the area of comprehension that emphasizes learning of strategies to understand text. Reading comprehension includes a student's ability to:

- Apply his or her knowledge and experiences to the text

- Draw inferences and logical conclusions from what is read

- Use strategies and skills to construct meaning from the written word

- Recognize the author's purpose

- Separate fact from opinion

- Understand cause and effect

- Adapt strategies to understand various types of text (e.g., fiction novel versus history textbook)

There are several standardized tests available to assess reading comprehension. Teachers can use these measures, along with their personal knowledge of student progress, to plan an appropriate program.

- Comprehensive Reading Assessment Battery (Fuchs, Fuchs, & Hamlett, 1989)

- Gates-MacGinitie Reading Tests (MacGinitie et al., 2000)

- Gray Oral Reading Test 4 (Wiederholt & Bryant, 2001)

- Gray Silent Reading Test (Wiederholt & Blalock, 2000)

- Test of Reading Comprehension (Brown et al., 1995)

- Standardized Reading Inventory 2 (Newcomer, 1999)

- Woodcock Reading Mastery (Woodcock, 1998)

The National Reading Panel's 2000 report suggested several strategies be used to enhance reading comprehension instruction. These were listed in Chapter 10.

While older children with VCFS typically can decode words fairly efficiently, the skills needed for success in reading in the upper elementary grades become much more difficult. Again, keeping in mind the deficits in working memory, it is logical that problems arise at this stage. Once a series of words are decoded a child needs to be able to hold the thought as the remainder of the paragraph is read. All of these thoughts must be remembered and stored as a page and then a chapter is deciphered. This task of keeping all of these thoughts in working memory becomes insurmountable and the result is a jumble of correctly decoded words, but poor comprehension and recall. Accommodations for this type of disability must center on methods of helping the child store or have access to as much of the information read as possible. Several techniques can be used to address this.

Before reading:

- Set a purpose for reading

- Teach key vocabulary

- Link student's background and experiences to story

- Relate the text to the student's life

- Survey the text for headings and pictures

- Predict what the story is about

- Make a KWL chart (student lists what he knows, what he wants to know, and what he learned after he reads in a chart format)

- Make a template to fill in with key story elements such as characters, setting, problem, rising action, climax, resolution

During reading:

- Guided reading: Use a fill-in-the-blank summary that a child completes as he or she reads the selection. Recording key information helps both with memory recall and with condensing the selection into more easily accessible notes.

- Oral reading of selection: Reading aloud helps the child to hear and see the text. This also improves comprehension and fluency. Students can read to the teacher, to themselves, or to a friend.

- Books on tape: Again, hearing the selection read with expression aids the comprehension of the selection. In the United States, students with disabilities are eligible to receive all of their texts on tape through services provided through their public library. They must register as a child with a disability, but once they do so they can receive this service through the Library of Congress program. If this service is not available, it may be possible for the school to provide tape recorded novels and texts.

- Use a tape recorder: Students can record the main idea of a selection as they read—perhaps at the end of a paragraph or page. They can then listen to this tape as they prepare to write a summary or book report.

■ Use templates: Students can use forms provided by the teacher to record important information as they read such as character names, setting, plot details, etc.

■ Reformat pages: Children with VCFS do better when pages are uncluttered and print is enlarged. Having fewer words on a page helps them focus and allows for easier visual tracking. Text read from a computer screen, rather than a printed page, can be helpful, also. If visual skills are impaired, other accommodations such as tilted work surfaces and colored filters to reduce glare might also be of assistance. Pages can also be scanned into the computer.

■ Use a structured reading program that builds from year to year: As mentioned in the section on reading in Chapter 10, students with learning difficulties need an approach that is organized around skill development. A clear understanding of the skills and objectives at each age level and a curriculum that builds in a linear fashion are necessary to offer consistency. Students in schools where teachers at different grade levels use vastly different approaches often miss critical skill development. When schools adopt a basal series, for example, and use the same program several successive years, there is a built-in scope and sequence for instruction. This incremental building of skills is preferred over the more global, whole language approach.

■ Teach students to monitor their understanding and to reread if necessary. Use modeling to demonstrate reading strategies.

■ Use small group literary circles where students can discuss the story with each other and clarify understanding.

■ Illustrate parts of the book.

After reading:

■ Complete the last part of KWL log (what I learned)

■ Reread notes and summarize main ideas

■ Answer teacher-generated questions

■ Complete a project such as a book jacket, poster, skit, diorama, etc.

■ Use flash cards to drill important information from reading needed for a test

■ Assess comprehension both in oral and written form with student

■ Consider reading shorter passages, rather than longer books, if student is struggling.

## MATHEMATICS

The subject of mathematics will likely continue to be very challenging for students with velo-cardio-facial syndrome. Almost all students report difficulty understanding the abstract concepts needed to successfully solve story problems. The relationship between language and math operations eludes them and they have a hard time translating word problems to mathematical equations. Equally as troubling is solving multistep problems, understanding geometric concepts, interpreting measurement relationships, or comprehending abstract applications. With repeated drill and practice students can learn to solve computational problems, do rote algebraic manipulations, or substitute numbers into given formulas. Their understanding, however, is usually limited to more rote memorization than real numerical insight. Hopefully, the suggestions in the earlier chapters will improve this situation for younger children. For many students, however, this impairment seems to persist despite various remediation attempts using numerous educational approaches. A large number of adults with VCFS report that they need assistance with budgeting, handling money, and understanding mathematical ideas. While the task seems somewhat daunting, reasonable math proficiency can be attained with this syndrome given persistence and practice.

The approaches to teaching math discussed in Chapter 10 are applicable to this level as well. Some additional suggestions for math educational approaches at upper elementary are discussed below.

Strong reinforcement of basic computational skills should continue to be taught. Although most typically developing students at this level have their addition and subtraction facts mastered, children with VCFS should continue to practice these skills to achieve instant recall. Again, this frees more brainpower to apply to problem solving and more complicated problems. It also gives these children, who often have a relative strength in memorization, an area of math they can reasonably master.

If at all possible, math facts should be memorized by the end of fourth grade (age 9+)—using music, flash cards, rhymes, index cards with troublesome facts posted around the room, and computer drill programs all help cement these facts into memory. Students will struggle in upper level courses without these facts mastered. For example, instruction in fractions, where numbers need to be simplified using factors, will be extremely challenging without knowledge of multiplication facts. Using a calculator can help somewhat but isn't a substitute for knowing factual relationships of numbers.

Use a direct instruction rather than a discovery approach to teaching math—math programs that use a discovery approach will be very difficult for children with VCFS who will likely not be able to see connections or logically reason through math strategies. A program that clearly demonstrates math concepts and provides a lot of practice with applications is preferable. If a spiraling curriculum is adopted, provide that the child is given many opportunities to learn a new concept. Many times a child with VCFS will need to redo a skill many more times than a typically developing child. Teaching the depth of a concept (such as spending several weeks or months learning fraction operations) is a better approach than trying to cover the concept quickly with the idea that it will be retaught later. The programs mentioned earlier, Number Worlds, On Cloud Nine math, Singapore Math, all have upper elementary components.

Use opportunities to teach concepts in real life situations. As stated earlier in the book, it is very helpful to teach math within the context of real life situations. Children with VCFS are usually concrete thinkers and have trouble relating to abstract or hypothetical book situations. Any time the math idea can be incorporated into a real life, hands-on experience will help with understanding. Adults working with the child can also try to reword story problems to include the names of familiar people or common experiences to which the child can relate.

Use graph paper to help visually—using graph paper is helpful to keep columns straight during calculations and to help organize work on the paper.

Keep the number of problems on a page to a minimum and enlarge print—resizing the print and eliminating clutter on the page will help accommodate for visual perceptual difficulties. It also will reduce the anxiety of a struggling child who is faced with many problems to solve on one page.

Eliminate the need to copy problems before solving them—if possible do not require the child with VCFS to recopy problems out of a book. Poor fine motor and copying skills make this task problematic. Let the child focus efforts on solving the math problem, not copying it.

Teach students to draw a picture of the math problem. Visually seeing the problem can aid in understanding. Use diagrams, formulas, and step-by-step approaches to solve more complex problems.

Remember to spend time on the vocabulary aspect of math. Children with VCFS have underlying language impairments. They will need direct instruction to understand the language of story problems and will need to learn key words to help them interpret the math operation(s) needed. For example, the words altogether, sum, or total all indicate addition. The key words more than, difference, or less than mean to subtract. They will need to understand the various uses of numbers, such as to quantify (5 books), label (124 King Street), locate (fourth on a line), and to measure (6 centimeters). They also will need continued instruction in interpreting different magnitude and number comparisons. The Thinker Math program by Carole Greenes, Linda Schulman, and Rika Spungin, available at http://www.wrightgroup.com, uses a fill-in-the-blank, story problem format to teach number sense and math language. Students read a short paragraph that has several blanks with missing numbers. Correct answers in random order are given in a box next to the paragraph. Students must fill in the blanks with the numbers that make sense within the context of the paragraph.

An example, from p. 15 for the grade 5–6 edition follows:

> The widest long-span bridge is the _____ foot long Sydney Harbor Bridge built in Australia in _____. The length of the bridge is about 10 times its width. The bridge is _____ feet wide. It has _____ railroad tracks, _____ lanes of roadway, a cycle way and a walkway. There are 4 times as many lanes of roadway as railroad tracks.
>
> Number choices for the blanks are: 160, 1932, 8, 2, and 1,650.

Finally, it is recommended that students use calculators to check work or to do more difficult, laborious calculations but not as a substitute for learning math facts or basic math algorithms. Once students are proficient with basic calculations, calculators are an appropriate tool to solve more advanced math problems. However, at this level, students should learn to be comfortable with 1- or 2-digit number operations and to do skills such as basic estimation, decimal/percent/fraction conversions (50% = 0.5 = ½), money conversions, measurement problems, etc., without the aid of a calculator.

## UPPER ELEMENTARY CONTENT AREAS OF SOCIAL STUDIES AND SCIENCE

Students in the upper elementary school are beginning to be held accountable for remembering facts, historical events, and scientific information. In the United States, the No Child Left Behind law has mandated that schools test students often for mastery of state standards. This movement will definitely impact what is taught in school and what students will need to master as they progress through the grades. Some states have stringent guidelines on the scores students will need on these tests in order to pass from one grade to the next. Because the topics of social studies and science are so broad, it is necessary to at least try to narrow the focus so that schools can adequately prepare students to succeed on these assessments. Many educators complain that their curriculum is now test-driven and that they are spending too much time "teaching to the test." This preparation for the exam, however, is extremely important for the child with VCFS. In all states, despite their educational disabilities, children with VCFS will be required to participate in this testing. It differs from state to state, however, how the results will be used. It is my hope that the results will be used as a template for remediation and not as a barrier to grade promotion or school graduation.

With that said, the focus on instruction in the content areas should center on a hands-on, experiential approach coupled with multiple opportunities to practice the skills identified in the unit. For exampled, well-planned lessons on invertebrates might look something like this:

Day 1:  Introduction to invertebrates: Have child *make* vocabulary note cards, *read out loud* with teacher or partner text information (one page max), *discuss* characteristics of sponges with child one-on-one to confirm understanding. *Play* game with vocabulary cards.

Day 2:  Activity to *draw* hollow-bodied animal and locate important body parts. Introduce hollow-bodied animals and point out differences and similarities. *Fill in* a Venn diagram to show differences. *Read* about sponges in textbook (out loud with child). *Discuss* topic with child. *Handle* a sponge specimen—look at parts under a microscope.

Day 3:  Introduce mollusks: Watch video (provide child with a written summary of main ideas and a guided fill-in-the-answer sheet). *Identify* parts of mollusks on a diagram. Have class *set up* several small aquariums with different numbers of snails and amounts of elodea or other aquatic plants. Observe over several days to determine which aquatic environment works the best. Have student *record* observations. Work one-on-one with the child with VCFS to help him or her understand the method behind setting up a scientific experiment. *Record* main idea, conclusion, etc., in a lab notebook.

The emphasis in all of these lessons is to have the child actively doing something measurable during class to enhance his or her understanding of the topic. It is also imperative that one-on-one instruction occurs to reinforce ideas and to check for understanding of content. It is also very helpful if lessons are simplified to emphasize the main concepts and that written study guides are provided to the child. Finally, parents or tutors need to review the study guides at home, several times per week, to insure better retention of material. Remember, in order for a child with VCFS to be able to retain learned information to use again, they will need to review and practice the concept multiple times. A one-time class presentation will not be sufficient for the child to master the lesson.

Some concepts can be successfully taught using a simulation approach. This works particularly well in the social studies area where history can be rather abstract and difficult to interpret. http//www.highsmith.com is a Web site selling units entitled Interact that allow students to role play historical situations. For example in one scenario, students take the role of a pioneer in the late 1840s traveling down the Oregon Trail. Each student gets a pioneer identity and has to make decisions regarding what supplies to take along and how to respond when unplanned challenges occur on the trip.

Money skills and economic concepts can be taught using a money simulation activity. Students at Elm Lawn Elementary School in Middleton, WI, look forward all year to the annual money unit that takes place the last quarter of the school year. Each student begins the unit with $500 in play money, a checking account, and a savings account. Students are paid $50 every two weeks and can earn additional money by selling goods that they produce at the weekly markets. They can also earn interest on the money they deposit in savings. Students can receive fines for late work, noise pollution, speeding (running in the hallways), etc. They also need to write out $10 rent checks (for their desks) every other week. The unit culminates with an auction for real goods the last day of school where students can bid on donated items using the money they have earned during the unit. This type of learning activity would help a child with VCFS put abstract ideas into a real life context. It would also allow practice with real life money skills in a meaningful, motivating way.

See lists in Appendix A for many more accommodation ideas.

## SOCIAL AND EMOTIONAL ISSUES AT UPPER ELEMENTARY GRADES

Upper elementary school is often a difficult time socially for students with disabilities. Students begin to solidify relationships and often groups of children begin excluding others from their friendship circles. In addition, children become quite busy with after-school sports or enrichment activities and their schedules leave little time for just "hanging out" at home with friends. In addition, these after-school activities become the basis for forming core friendship groups, and students that do not participate are left out of the loop.

Children with VCFS often have trouble excelling in typical group sports activities. Many still have issues with low muscle tone, poor eye-hand coordination, balance, and attention. In addition, their after-school time may be spent in tutoring sessions, at medical appointments, or with various therapists. Therefore, their primary social contacts tend to be with adults rather than other children.

While it certainly is important that children with VCFS get the remediation and medical help they need, it is also imperative that time is set aside for participation is some type of after-school activity involving other children. A caring adult who can help the child with VCFS learn appropriate social behavior should also monitor the activity. Sports activities that are less competitive are probably also a better choice. Philosophies that promote inclusion of all participants are preferable.

Some children with VCFS have had success with dance team activities, karate/martial arts training, or gymnastics experiences. Memorizing gross motor moves seems to be easier for many than remembering written facts. These activities can also improve motor skills, balance, listening, and remembering verbal directions. Other options to explore are scouting activities, clubs through the child's church or synagogue, or after-school activities programs.

Finally, it is interesting to note that a great number of children with VCFS seem to be able to develop a talent for music. It is unclear just why musical skill comes easier for this population, but casual data collected of children with VCFS supports this. Despite having a great deal of difficulty learning academic skills, playing drums, guitar, or piano comes more naturally.

When considering music lessons, keep in mind the unique learning needs of children with VCFS and try to find a teacher willing to work in a different manner. Try to avoid a program with heavy emphasis on sight-reading and music theory. Instead opt for a looser, less academic approach. Remember the goal of the music training is to nurture a talent that the child might rely on later in life for a social outlet. Young adults can find a lot of enjoyment and opportunities for friendships if they can play an instrument well enough to join a casual band. Most importantly, try not to nag the child to practice. Many children with VCFS love playing music in a relaxing nonpressured atmosphere.

If friendship problems do develop, do not ignore the problems. Children who are ignored or teased at school are at greater risk for depression. Given the high rate of psychiatric problems in the VCFS population, it is imperative that a carefully planned program to enhance self-esteem and lower environmental stressors is warranted. Schools can institute friendship programs, bullying prevention curriculums, and social skills training. The staff can also assist with activities that celebrate differences and promote the acceptance of inclusion for students with disabilities. All students need to feel that they have at least one friend that they can socialize with throughout the school day—especially at lunch and recess times. Teachers and counselors can facilitate friendships by hosting lunchtime friendship groups or assisting with small group friendship circles. In the classroom, teachers can try to pair up the students with VCFS with other children with similar interests. In any case, adults need to realize they may have to take a more active role than usual to promote healthy social development with students with VCFS.

## LIFE SKILLS

Typical curriculums for students of this age do not include a lot of direct instruction in life skills. It is assumed that these skills are learned through everyday experiences or at home. For example, students learn shopping skills, cooking, grooming, money, and time concepts from day-to-day life interactions. Unfortunately, students with VCFS often need more intense instruction in these areas. Attainment Company specializes in software and educational materials that target students with special needs who need to have a formal curriculum in life skills. The company, located in Verona, Wisconsin, can be accessed at http://www.AttainmentCompany.com. Many of the materials offered require only basic reading skills and they cover a wide variety of practical needs. Parents can also order these materials for use at home with their child to reinforce these necessary independent living skills.

## REFERENCES

Broadley, I. W., & MacDonald, J. (1993). Teaching short term memory skills to children with Down syndrome. *Down Syndrome Research and Practice, 1*, 56–62.

Broadley, I., MacDonald, J., & Buckley, S. (1999). Working memory in children with Down syndrome. *Down Syndrome Research and Practice, 3* (1), 3–8.

Brown, V., Hammill, J., & Wiederholt, L. (1995). *Test of reading comprehension.* Austin, TX: Pro-Ed.

Butler, R., & Copeland, D. (2002). Attentional processes and their remediation in children treated for cancer: A literature review and the development of a therapeutic approach, *Journal of the International Neuropsychological Society, 8*, 115–124.

Fuchs, L., Fuch, D. & Hamlett. (1989). In monitoring growth using student recall: Effects of two teacher feedback systems. *Journal of Educational Research, 83*(2), 103–111.

Greenes, C., Schulman, L., & Spungin, R. (1989). *Thinker math, developing number sense and arithmetic skills.* Mountain View, CA: Creative Publications.

Klingberg, T., Fernell, E., Olesen, P., Johnson, M., Gustafsson, P., Dahlstrom, K., et al. (2005). Computerized training of working memory in children with ADHD—A randomized, controlled trial. *Journal of American Academy of Child and Adolescent Psychiatry, 44* (2), 177–186.

MacGinitie, W., MacGinitie, R., Maria, K., Dreyer, L., & Hughes, K. (2000). *Gates-MacGinitie Reading Tests.* Rolling Meadows, IL: Riverside.

Newcomer, P. (1999). *Standardized Reading Inventory 2.* Austin, TX: Pro-Ed.

Olesen, P., Westerberg, H., & Klingberg, T. (2004). Increased prefrontal and parietal activity after training of working memory. *Nature Neuroscience, 7*(1), 75–79.

Stevenson, C., Whitmont, S., Bornholt, L., Livesay, D., & Stevenson, R. (2002). A cognitive remediation programme for adults with attention deficit hyperactivity disorder, *Australian and New Zealand Journal of Psychiatry, 36*, 610–616.

Wiederholt J., Bryant, B. (2001). *Gray Oral Reading Test 4.* Austin, TX: Pro-Ed.

Wiederholt J., Blalack, B.. (2000). *Gray Silent Reading Test.* Austin, TX: Pro-Ed.

Woodcock, R. (1998). *Woodcock Reading Mastery.* Bloomington, MN: Pearson Assessments.

Wykes, T., Brammer, M., Mellers, J., Bray, P., Reeder, C., Williams, C., et al. (2002). Effects on the brain of a psychological treatment: Cognitive remediation therapy. Functional magnetic resonance imaging in schizophrenia. *British Journal of Psychiatry, 181*, 144–152.

Wykes, T., Reeder, C., Corner, J., Williams, C., & Everitt, B. (1999). The effects of neurocognitive remediation on executive processing in patients with schizophrenia. *Schizophrenia Bulletin, 25*, 291–308.

■ Additional services were provided in speech and language therapy, which addressed advocacy skills, communication deficits, job application/interview skills, etc.

■ A vision specialist helped with visual perceptual training and with providing necessary supports.

■ The student enrolled in one class first semester and two classes second semester at the local technical college. The case manager, provided by the school district, helped the student with the class assignments. The case manager also assisted by contacting instructors to clarify assignments and help with enrollment and accessing disability services. The tuition for these classes was provided by the school district.

■ The student worked as an assistant at a local karate school. The school district worked to help the VCFS student understand his job responsibilities, keep appointments, react appropriately to situations related to his work, plan his schedule, and understand how to read his pay stub.

■ The case manager put together a binder with all necessary phone numbers and contacts the student would need in case of an emergency. A budget and plan for independent living were also drafted and the student began to look for a place to live away from home.

■ Plans were made for a vocational assessment (paid for by the Department of Vocational Rehabilitation) to be done the next summer.

■ Connections were put in place for eventual transfer to the Developmental Disabilities Department for adult state programs and the parents applied for supplemental Social Security benefits on their child's behalf.

The second year of the program:

■ Continued support with daily living skills provided at the district administrative center by the case manager.

■ Continued enrollment at the local technical college in the small business program (two classes completed first semester, three second).

■ Tutoring help provided by the school district.

■ Job exploration opportunities including job shadowing and vocational assessments.

■ Job support with the karate school job placement including adding additional responsibilities at the school. Continued training in karate skills, which will lead to a third degree black belt before the end of the year.

- Leadership training (offered through karate school) to train potential lead instructors—this would be a better paying position with benefits.

- Help with independent living skills at an apartment student shared with another adult.

- Continued help with budgeting, organization, managing medication, and other life skills (provided by school district case manager).

- In the spring, coordination with the Developmental Disabilities State Program to have a case manager in place when student graduates in June (he will be 21) to assume responsibilities for job coaching and life skill support.

- Coordination with the Department of Vocational Rehabilitation to continue to support the student at the technical college as he completes the credits he needs for a small business diploma.

At the time of graduation at age 21, this student made great progress toward his goal of independent living and job placement. He was much better prepared to attend technical college independently to complete his degree. He will still need a lot of tutoring support and accommodations at the tech school, but he has a much better chance of succeeding. He has worked consistently at a job and made growth in his interpersonal relationships. He better understands the demands of an employer and has learned some organizational strategies. He has even, on occasion, taken over teaching a karate class independently. In addition because of the school supports, he has lived for several months at an apartment away from his parents, grocery shopped by himself, paid his own rent on time, managed his laundry, and kept his own schedule. Finally, he has gained self-confidence and a sense of purpose. He feels he has a plan for his life and that is both comforting and reassuring.

## APPLYING FOR COMMUNITY SUPPORTS

As stated earlier, a child who reaches the age of 18 is considered an adult in the United States and is eligible to apply for adult services. The rules vary from country to country, but most societies do assist their adult disabled population in some way. Adults with VCFS often do qualify for some type of adult help. Parents will need to investigate the criteria necessary for securing these services and for setting up their finances to properly care for their child.

The programs available in the United States include Social Security benefits, Department of Vocational Rehabilitation Assistance, and state-run programs for the disabled population. At the age of 18, a young adult with VCFS can apply for Supplemental Security Income (SSI) through the Social Security Administration (http://ssa.gov). There are numerous rules that govern this need-based program. For example, young adults are allowed to have no more than $2,000 in countable assets, they can earn a very limited monthly income, and they may not receive any assistance from others for food, clothing, or shelter. There is an application process to go through for a person to qualify as disabled under Social Security and often this can take several months. If a person qualifies, they will receive monthly checks to pay for living expenses, and most importantly he or she will qualify for health insurance through Medicaid. This is particularly important to consider because often a parent's health insurance will not pay for a child after the age of 18 if he or she is not a full-time student. Other policies pay until age 22 or 23 and then it is assumed that young adults will be employed and offered health insurance as a benefit or that they will be able to buy their own insurance. Young adults with VCFS will have a lot of difficulty finding health insurance they can afford because of their complicated medical histories and expensive medication requirements.

A good transition program will provide families with help securing resources in the community. Schools often can act as facilitators in helping families gather needed information and setting up meetings between the families and community supports. Young adults with VCFS and their families should not be expected to acquire these resources on their own. It is important that schools provide this service so that the transition to adult services is seamless and coordinated. In many communities, there are long waiting lists for services. Early planning is crucial to eliminate wasted years waiting for assistance with areas such as job coaching and work skill development. The IDEA law in the United States requires that transition planning begin as early as age 14. States have their own laws governing how they allocate community resources to the disabled populations. Educators at the high school level must become knowledgeable about these rules so that important deadlines are met, needed contacts are made, and paperwork is completed. In addition, most state agencies have not dealt with clients diagnosed with velo-cardio-facial syndrome. It is imperative that information about this syndrome and its impact on independent functioning be disseminated to the community.

## COLLEGE AND POST-SECONDARY TRAINING

For some young adults with VCFS and other developmental disabilities, college is an appropriate goal. A few adults with VCFS have completed four-year college programs and are employed as educators or in other professions.

Colleges with strong disability resource services are preferable. It is also necessary for the young adult to be willing and able to seek help from these centers. Hiring a tutor is recommended, as is monitoring of work completion deadlines and exam schedules.

College is stressful for all students. The demands are heavy. The workload is intense, professors are less willing to modify expectations, and the course content is complicated. Students who live away from home have the added pressures of successfully coping with roommates or dorm/apartment life. Students with VCFS have the added vulnerability to mental health issues that may intensify in their late teens and early twenties. Stress can exacerbate symptoms, so care should be taken to assure that the work expectations and living situation are appropriate.

The transition model discussed earlier allowed for a college experience with a net of support from the high school and later from community agencies. A light course load, daily tutoring, support with living skills, and strong family support made this a successful experience. Many communities have college programs that are less intense than a four-year academically challenging university. These schools offer a wide variety of diploma programs such as small business ownership, recreation management, nursing assistant, etc. They also provide training in apprentice careers like carpentry, plumbing, auto repair, and culinary arts. Young adults with VCFS will need help sorting out a program that is both interesting and manageable.

Finally, it is worth noting that enrollment in a post-secondary program has benefits beyond just the course content. It allows young adults an opportunity to socialize with others their own age, move about on a college campus, advocate for themselves in a new environment, and gain a sense of accomplishment. Furthermore, it gives them a purpose to their day and helps them have a positive outlook to the future. A wide variety of training programs do exist and educators should consider counseling families on the possibilities available.

## BIBLIOGRAPHY/SUGGESTED READINGS

Crawford, V., & Silver, L. B. (2002). *Embracing the monster: Overcoming the challenges of hidden disabilities.* Baltimore: P. H. Brookes.

Crux, S. C. (1991). *Learning strategies for adults: Compensations for learning disabilities.* Toronto: Wall & Emerson.

Fast, Y. (2004). *Employment for individuals with Asperger syndrome or non-verbal learning disability: Stories and strategies.* London: Jessica Kingsley.

Levinson, E. (2004). *Transition from school to post school life for individuals with disabilities, Assessment from an educational and school psychological perspective.* Springfield, IL: Thomas.

Mooney, J., & Cole, D. (2000). *Learning outside the lines: Two Ivy League students with learning disabilities and ADHD give you the tools for academic success and educational revolution.* New York: Simon & Schuster.

Nadeau, K. G. (1994). *Survival guide for college students with ADD or LD*. New York: Magination Press.

Palmer, A. (2006). *Realizing the college dream with autism or Asperger syndrome: A parent's guide to student success*. London: Jessica Kingsley.

Patton, J. R., & Polloway, E. A. (1996). *Learning disabilities: The challenges of adulthood*. Austin, TX: Pro-Ed.

Pierangelo, R., & Crane, R. (1997). *Complete guide to special education transition services: Ready to use guide for successful transitions from school to adulthood*. Allyn & Bacon.

Pierangelo, R., & Giulani, G. (2003). *Transition services in special education: A practical approach*. Upper Saddle River, NJ: Allyn & Bacon.

Quinn, P. O. (1994). *ADD and the college student: A guide for high school and college students with attention deficit disorder*. Washington, DC: Magination Press.

Richer, S., & Weir, L. (1995). *Beyond political correctness: Toward the inclusive university*. Buffalo, NY: University of Toronto Press.

Sitlington, P., & Clark, G. (2005). *Transition education and services for students with disabilities*. Upper Saddle River, NJ: Allyn & Bacon.

Wehman, P. (2006). *Life beyond the classroom, Transition strategies for young people with disabilities*. Baltimore: P. H. Brookes.

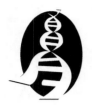

# Conclusion

*T*here are many reasons to be optimistic about the future for students with VCFS. Scientific studies to understand the reasons behind the learning and behavioral difficulties with VCFS are more abundant, and interest in the syndrome has increased tremendously. Pharmacological treatments for attention, memory, and mental health disabilities are improving and studies are underway to test how these treatments affect the VCFS population. As more research is completed, interventions specifically targeted to children with VCFS will be better tailored to meet their needs. The challenge now is to formally assess the efficacy of the interventions attempted. Hopefully, in the meantime this book will provide a template for educators to design more effective interventions. At the very least, it will serve as a handbook to familiarize professionals with the unique needs of the VCFS population.

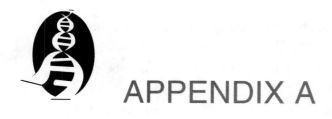

# APPENDIX A

# Accommodations

## ACADEMIC DELAYS

- Write key points on the board prior to or during lecture
- Allow more time to process information (speak more slowly, give more "wait time")
- Have student verbally summarize key points throughout the lesson to check comprehension of the material
- Break longer presentations into shorter parts
- Provide more modeling, demonstration, and guided practice
- Provide many opportunities to verbalize in class reinforcing the student's willingness to participate, even if the answer is not correct
- Have the student or another student repeat directions/instructions to check comprehension
- Preview textbook or handouts for each unit with student
- Provide extra time to read material
- Preteach vocabulary/concepts for each unit
- Read textbook in class or in pairs
- Use computer for word processing written work
- Provide easy to read handouts, free of clutter and extra wording

■ Provide immediate feedback regarding newly taught skill and reteach concepts not learned

■ Check within the first few minutes of an assignment to be sure student is doing the work correctly

■ Allow student to use learning aide (i.e., computerized spell checker, calculator, reading markers, audio tapes, charts, number lines, etc.)

■ Allow student to dictate answers to someone: parent, aide, etc.

## ORGANIZATION OF ASSIGNMENTS

■ Allow extra time for finishing assignments

■ Provide a timeline for completing portions of long-term assignments

■ Set short-term goals for work completion

■ Provide direct instruction on organization skills

■ Post assignments and due dates in a prominent place in the room

■ Use and monitor assignment notebook daily

■ Have an aide or teacher recheck the assignment notebook and help student gather needed materials to take home

■ Provide students with handouts that are three-hole punched and use this type of binder

■ Use an accordion folder with subject dividers to keep loose papers organized

■ Remind students of assignments orally and visually at the end of the period and cue them to record them in assignment books

■ Color-code books, notebooks, and materials by subject area

■ Tape "Things to Do" list to student's desk or notebook

■ Have a set time and place for student to hand in assignments

■ Allow student some leniency on late work

■ Reduce clutter in locker and student's desk

■ Pair students to check work

■ Shorten assignment or break it into smaller parts

■ At home: set aside a study area with all necessary materials handy and have a homework time scheduled daily

## EVALUATIONS AND TESTING

■ Allow student to demonstrate knowledge through projects or presentations

■ Mark student's correct work, not the mistakes

■ Allow extra time for taking/completing tests

■ Allow student to have test read and interpreted to him or her

■ Alter type of examination (i.e., portfolio, authentic, and performance assessments)

■ Allow open book and open note exams

■ Put the test on audio cassette

■ Give take-home tests

■ Use computer assisted instructional evaluations

■ Allow test retakes

■ Allow student to dictate test answers

■ Provide pretest and posttest

■ Give students a concise study guide

■ Provide an alternative to Scantron (fill in the dot) computerized sheets

## TEST WRITING

■ Give fewer choices on multiple-choice tests

■ Provide word banks for all short answer, essay, and fill-in-the-blank tests

■ Develop test questions and directions using simple, direct vocabulary and grammar

■ On matching sections of tests, break into five to seven items per section

- On matching portions of tests, put the longer, definition part on the left and the vocabulary word on the right

- Provide direct instruction on how to take different types of tests (i.e., strategies for multiple test taking, use part of the question in the answer for essays)

- Give several tests over a relatively small amount of material, rather than one test over a lot of information

- Break test into two parts and give over two days

- Avoid pop quizzes

- Provide a template form for essay answers and allow the use of a word processor

## HOME/SCHOOL COMMUNICATION

- Provide positive daily rewards for bringing completed assignments, assignment books, and/or progress notes home

- Set up daily/weekly communications to be signed by parent and teacher

- Increase phone contact between school and home, remembering to share positive information as well as concerns

- Schedule more frequent conferences

- Obtain resources to better understand student's impairments

## HANDWRITING AND FINE/VISUAL MOTOR ACCOMMODATIONS

- Allow student to write on larger paper with clearly marked lines for guides

- Provide graph paper for math calculations

- Allow the student to use a word processor for written work

- Allow student to use a variety of fine motor aids such as thick pencils, felt tip pens, pencil grips, special scissors, etc.

- Provide student with a sample page of what you want the paper to look like

- Attach the paper to a clipboard or slant board to keep paper stable while working

- Grade handwriting separate from language

- Highlight margins and starting or ending points for sentences

- Allow student extra time for written assignments

- Reduce written requirements (e.g., do not make students copy math problems)

- Allow student to tape record or dictate answers

- Allow student to copy peer's notes or use a note taker

- Check student's sitting posture and help make adjustments

- Do not make student copy from board, but rather provide information on a piece of paper

- Allow student to use a computer for essay tests or for other written work

## PHYSICAL ARRANGEMENT OF THE ROOM/CLASSROOM ENVIRONMENT

- Seat student near teacher

- Seat student near a positive role model and well-focused students

- Stand near the student when giving directions

- Use an FM system

- Increase distance between students' desks

- Provide quiet areas with a study carrel to minimize distractions

- Reduce clutter around the room and at student's desk

- Clearly mark locations of materials and supplies

- Post daily schedule or tape schedule to student's desk/notebook

- Seat student away from distractions (i.e., door, windows, high traffic areas)

- Allow student frequent breaks to move around
- Allow student to use sensorimotor techniques in the classroom to regulate him- or herself including eating, chewing, etc.
- Provide appropriate sized furniture
- Provide access to sensory room in school to do larger motor activities
- Use colors or light changes to help with regulation
- Provide computer access
- Limit class size and provide for one-on-one or small group work periods

## NOTETAKING

- Provide note taker or have a peer use carbon paper to copy notes
- Provide written outline or study guide
- Allow student to tape record review sessions or lectures
- Provide student with computer presentations
- Provide student with a partially completed outline or classroom notes omitting key words for student to fill in
- Provide summary of videos
- Provide student with highlighted textbook

## WORKING MEMORY ACCOMMODATIONS

- Allow student to use notes on tests
- Teach memory techniques
- Use reminder lists
- Use an assignment notebook and calendar
- Post assignments prominently in classroom
- Verbally cue student to help him or her remember

- Use word banks on assignments or tests
- Keep classroom organized—assign places for supplies, books, etc.
- Have students write really important reminders in washable marker on his/her hand
- Color code folders by subject
- Teach student to file papers in the proper place immediately after finishing them
- Use accordion folders with subject dividers to keep papers
- Use mnemonics to help students remember information
- Have students study in short chunks over several days rather than in one long session
- Allow open book tests
- Use drill and practice with multiple repetitions to help memory storage
- Revisit earlier learned skills several times during the school year to help with recall

## BEHAVIOR ACCOMMODATIONS

- Prepare students for changes in routines
- Clearly define procedures/rules for daily routines (i.e., bathroom breaks, use of computers, independent work time, how to ask for help, etc.)
- Delay instruction until it is quiet and students are attending (use cues like turn off light, ring bell, raise hand)
- Use music during transitions and for calming student
- Provide frequent breaks and opportunities to move
- Give frequent feedback and progress checks for academic work
- Provide private, personal cuing signals for student
- Provide contract/behavior program for specific behaviors; include positive reinforcement/rewards (phone calls, extra rewards or privileges, special activities, etc.)
- Reinforce behaviors frequently

- Allow student to determine consequences and reward for behavior
- Use self-regulation techniques
- Anticipate problems and use preventative strategies
- Ignore minor inappropriate behaviors
- Teach peers to ignore minor inappropriate behaviors
- Provide assistance during transition times
- Look for signs of stress and if necessary provide help or reduce work
- Allow student opportunity to "save face"
- Teach self-control and model appropriate behavior (i.e., walk away, use calming strategies)
- Find opportunities for student to display leadership/expertise in class
- Give student choices
- Handle teasing and bullying firmly on a schoolwide basis
- Reinforce student frequently when student is frustrated
- Be flexible with grading and encourage student to put forth best effort
- Stand close by student and provide assistance when necessary
- Provide an aide in the classroom to assist student
- Allow student to leave the room and go to the sensory room to calm down and refocus
- Use daily/weekly communication with home to monitor behavior progress
- Seek assistance from school counselor or school psychologist if behavior difficulties escalate or seem very unusual

## ACCOMMODATION FOR STUDENTS WITH NONVERBAL LEARNING DISABILITIES

- Observe the child across situations that are unstructured, novel, or complex. Focus on what the child does rather than what the child says.
- Teach in a structured step-by-step fashion. Provide verbal cues and information. Beware that concepts involving time, numbers, and magnitude will be particularly difficult.

■ Have student try to describe the details of important directions or learning concepts and clarify discrepancies or misconceptions if they exist.

■ Teach the child appropriate strategies for dealing with problems on a day-to-day basis. Do not assume child will be able to problem-solve independently. Videotaping may help point out appropriate behavior.

■ Help the student generalize learned concepts

■ If an older child is unable to grasp basic skills provide tools to help such as calculators, memory notebooks, navigation systems, digital clocks, locks without dials, timers, etc.

■ Teach social conversation skills such as what to say, how to say it, when to make a comment, etc.

■ Allow extra time for tests.

■ Help with handwriting practice, but allow word-processed assignments.

■ Give direct instruction in how to focus and attend to visual details.

■ Provide objects child can manipulate to help visualize math concepts.

■ If the student is impulsive, have him or her use the process of stop, look, listen, and weigh alternatives to behavior. Teach child to think about consequences.

■ Teach mechanical arithmetic in a step-by-step verbal and written fashion.

■ Use an assignment notebook or organizing system in elementary school, so it becomes more a routine habit by middle school.

■ Teach in shortened periods and allow frequent breaks.

■ Minimize visual distractions.

■ Teach child to recognize nonverbal cues and to link these with understanding others' feelings and intentions.

■ Present information in plain language and relate it to a familiar situation. Don't expect the child to grasp abstract meanings to "read between the lines."

■ Tasks involving folding, cutting, using tools may be troublesome, so plan to provide assistance.

■ Provide a predictable schedule.

■ Provide assistance and verbal/written cues to locations of places.

■ Help child organize his or her desk and locker.

■ Identify a case manager at school to oversee the student's progress, monitor implementation of accommodations, connect the school to home, and become the staff person the student seeks for assistance.

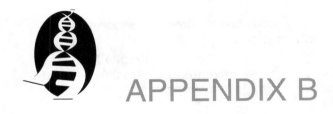

# APPENDIX B

# Teacher Awareness Questionnaire (Answers)

## TEACHER AWARENESS QUESTIONNAIRE
### (MARKS OF AN "X" ARE CORRECT)

Please indicate which of the following *cognitive features* are associated with each disorder (*Check all that apply*):

| | Down syndrome | Fragile X (male) | VCFS |
|---|---|---|---|
| Arithmetic as a relative weakness, below IQ level | | X | X |
| Relative strength in verbal-based learning | | X | X |
| Ave IQ 70 | | | X |
| Ave IQ 60 | X | | |
| Ave IQ 50 | | X | |
| Deficit in grammar/syntax | X | X | |
| Short-term memory deficit | X | X | X |
| Perseveration on word, thought, or task | X | X | X |
| Sequencing deficit | X | X | X |
| Expressive language stronger than receptive language (Ability to speak stronger than ability to understand) | | | X |

Please indicate which of the following *behavioral features* are associated with each disorder (*Mark with an "X" all that apply*):

| | Down syndrome | Fragile X (male) | VCFS |
|---|:---:|:---:|:---:|
| **Attention deficit/hyperactivity** | X | X | X |
| **Hypernasal speech** | | | X |
| **Gaze avoidance** | | X | |
| **Depression** | X | X | X |
| **Anxiety** | X | X | X |
| **Relative preservation of social skills** | X | | |
| **Schizophrenia/bipolar disorder** | | | X |
| **Multiple autistic-like features** | | | |
| **General happy temperament** | X | | |
| **Tactile defensiveness** | | X | |

Please indicate which of the following *physical features* are associated with each disorder (*Mark with an "X" all that apply*):

| | Down syndrome | Fragile X (male) | VCFS |
|---|:---:|:---:|:---:|
| **Large or prominent ears** | | X | |
| **Vision impairments** | X | X | X |
| **Cleft palate** | | | X |
| **Delayed motor development** | X | X | X |
| **Upslanting eyes** | X | | |
| **Hearing problems/deficits** | | X | X |

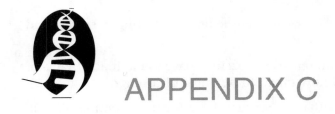

## APPENDIX C

# Exercises for Understanding

*T*he following questions and scenarios are designed to help educators dialog and plan for a child with VCFS. Many of the situations are drawn from actual IEP meetings or discussions that have occurred in schools around the world.

### PART 1: UNDERSTANDING THE VCFS SYNDROME

1. How would you describe velo-cardio-facial syndrome to educators?

2. Is there a difference between velo-cardio-facial syndrome, 22q11 deletion syndrome, and DiGeorge syndrome?

3. How is a child diagnosed with VCFS?

4. What medical clues might alert a professional that a child may have VCFS?

5. What subtle physical characteristics are found in many children with VCFS?

6. What is the "typical" learning profile of VCFS students and is this true of all students with the syndrome?

7. How does VCFS differ from fragile X and Down syndrome?

8. Given the neurocognitive research results reported in Chapter 2, what are the inconsistencies in the data?

9. What data have been consistent across the many studies discussed?

10. What is the difference between neurocognitive testing research and brain imaging studies?

11. What are some of the differences researchers have found in the brains of children with VCFS and how might these impact learning?

12. What are some theories that researchers have for the attention difficulties found with the syndrome?

13. What are further areas of study that you think researchers should pursue?

14. What language impairments do children with VCFS have and how does this change as the child matures?

15. What articulation difficulties do children with VCFS have and how are they treated?

16. What are the more common medical difficulties associated with VCFS and how might these affect school performance?

17. Where are the leading centers around the world studying VCFS located and how could you access additional information about the syndrome?

18. Describe some of the more common behavioral challenges that occur with VCFS.

19. What visual/spatial difficulties are associated with the syndrome and how might these affect a student with VCFS?

20. What is a nonverbal learning disability, and how is this related to VCFS?

21. What challenges do many teenagers and young adults with VCFS face and how might schools better meet their needs?

## PART 2: PLANNING AN EDUCATIONAL PROGRAM

1. Young children with VCFS have many needs. Given the timeline for interventions in Chapter 2, prioritize and design a program for the following preschool students with VCFS. Discuss the amount of time you would allocate for each intervention and why.

   Student 1:
   Kali is a 4½-year-old child with VCFS who has qualified for speech and language support. She has severe articulation difficulties and is barely understood by her parents and playmates. She often uses gestures rather than words in order to communicate and she is easily frustrated when her needs are not met. She engages in parallel play at school and other students complain that she doesn't share the toys. She has difficulty at drop-off time and often cries

for several minutes when her mother leaves in the morning. She has trouble handling the school supplies and often needs help completing any craft project. During large group time she loses interest after several minutes and at times she can disrupt the class activities. She enjoys listening to books and the teacher has noticed that Kali can recognize some printed words and can match them to the appropriate pictures. She is due to begin kindergarten next school year and the parents are concerned about her readiness for school.

Student 2:
Mark is a 4-year-old boy with VCFS. He has a ventricular septal heart defect that is small and has not required surgery. He has received speech and language intervention since he was 2 and also had surgery to help correct his hypernasal speech and articulation difficulties. He continues to sound different from other children and he is often teased about this issue. He tends to talk in short sentences with a limited vocabulary, but he is mostly understood by others. He is immature for his age, but separates fairly easily to attend preschool. Mark has hypotonia and has difficulty with handling school supplies, tying his shoes, and buttoning his clothes. He has chronic ear infections and has had surgery twice to place in ear tubes. He has a mild hearing loss. Mark follows the routine of the school day and especially enjoys reading and music. He can read several beginning books along with many signs posted around the classroom. He can count to 20, knows the alphabet, and has memorized several songs. He has a March birthday and his parents are also concerned about his readiness for school.

2. The following scenarios occurred with young children with VCFS in the United States. How would you handle the situations and plan more effectively for these youngsters?

Student 1:
Britta is a second grade girl with VCFS who has just this year transferred into a new school district. She receives speech and language support for 30 minutes twice a week from the special education department for articulation and language delays. Her FSIQ is 82 and tests indicate a higher verbal than performance IQ. Her first grade teacher reported that she was learning at a slower pace than the other students, but that she was making steady progress. She is reading at middle first grade level and her written language skills are at grade level. She struggles most with math and she is easily frustrated with the material. Her mother works with her at home, but reports that Britta often breaks down crying and

has said on several occasions that she hates math and that she is stupid. Britta has trouble staying focused for long periods of time and frequently comes home without the necessary papers to complete her work. Britta's teacher reports that Britta's behavior has deteriorated since the beginning of the school year. She pinches or hits other students and when asked she doesn't explain why she is upset. She has been placed on in-school suspension twice for her behavior and the principal is threatening to send Britta home for three days for the next conduct violation. Britta's mother is angry with the school for punishing her daughter, but the school insists it must insure the safety of the other students.

Student 2:
Scott is a second grade student with VCFS in a southern U.S. school district. His FSIQ is 83 and he has a documented speech and language disability. He receives resource room help 20 minutes per day and speech and language support twice a week for 30 minutes. His school's program is heavily dictated by the state standards for achievement. All children, regardless of ability, are required to complete the same curriculum, at the same pace. Scott was able to keep up with the others in his class last year, but this year the curriculum has become much more difficult for him. He is required to take tests over packets of materials in social studies and science that overwhelm him. After the first grading period, he was failing math, reading, science, and social studies. The only class he was passing was language arts. Scott consistently comes home with papers full of red marks and failing grades. His mother and father study with him every night at home and report that he seems to know the material when they review, but that he can't seem to perform on the tests. He cries many mornings before school and his parents are very concerned about his self-esteem. The school has offered to place him in a pull-out program for cognitively disabled students, but his parents want to keep him in the regular education program. They feel he has the potential to learn, but that he is not getting the appropriate interventions at school. The regular education teacher has a class size of 25 students and feels she is doing the best that she can.

3. Many students with VCFS have articulation/language difficulties that interfere with their ability to make friends and use pragmatic language effectively. Design a program to address this issue for an elementary school student.

4. Many children with VCFS are mainstreamed into the regular education program. Take a unit in science and social studies and modify it to better meet the needs of a child with the syndrome. Consider the classroom

environment, visual format of the written pages, the required memorization of terms, the vocabulary, the format of the assessment, the language needed to complete the lessons, and any other issues you think are relevant.

5. Math seems to be consistently difficult for students with VCFS. Look over various math curriculums and select a program that you think would work well and another program that you think would not. Compare the two programs and justify your decision.

6. Suppose your school district selected the program you feel would be least effective for use with a student with VCFS. Take a chapter from that program and modify it to better meet your student's needs.

7. John is a middle school student with VCFS. He has a mild hearing loss, low average cognitive ability, memory difficulties, language delay, and ADD. He receives special education support in the resource room. Despite his challenges, he makes good grades in his academic classes and works hard to succeed. He is, however, failing his physical education class. He cannot pass the written tests over the rules for the team sports the class has been studying, he seems lost in class, and he often does not dress in his gym clothes. What do you think might be causing the difficulties in this class and how can they be addressed?

8. What orientation program should a middle or high school provide for a student with visual/perceptual difficulties? What could the school do to help this student navigate the hallways, use the lockers, follow a schedule, etc.?

9. Discuss the pros and cons to a student with VCFS learning to drive. What criteria would you use to decide if this is a good decision?

10. Many high school classes involve a lecture format or cooperative learning groups. Both of these methods pose problems for students with VCFS. Receptive language difficulties make sitting through lectures ineffective. Cooperative learning groups have the potential to cause resentment from peers who are more efficient learners. There is also the risk that students with VCFS will learn very little if others do the bulk of the work. Discuss ways that students with VCFS can be fully included in high school classes at a level that insures their learning of the curriculum.

11. One of the major challenges facing educators working with a child with VCFS is being able to determine whether a particular intervention or strategy is effective. Design a prototype of an ongoing assessment method that you would use to determine if your student is learning at an acceptable pace. Use both curriculum-based assessment and curriculum-based measurement methods. In addition, develop a workable system for collecting the data and graphing your results.

12. Many students with genetic syndromes have difficulty focusing attention in a regular education classroom. Given the information on the weaknesses children with VCFS usually exhibit, how would you arrange the classroom environment to best meet their needs? Some factors you might consider are: desk arrangement, lighting, noise, written signs, use of a chalkboard, use of an overhead, materials around the room for student use, learning groups, etc.

13. Students with learning difficulties will likely need the support of family or after-school tutors to assist them with their academics. Role play how you would address this issue with parents who feel it is the school's responsibility to educate their child.

14. Many students with disabilities would benefit from a study guide to accompany a curriculum unit. Take a unit from the regular curriculum and devise a study guide to complement it. Include a calendar to help the student plan out study time in a way that would maximize the retention of the material. Pay special attention to formatting the pages in an uncluttered, inviting way.

15. Many students with VCFS can successfully be taught to calculate and apply mathematical formulas in a predictable way. Take a concept in mathematics (for example, area formulas in a measurement unit) and design templates this student can use to help understand the formulas. Experiment with color coding parts of the equations, enlarging the print, and simplifying the instruction methods.

16. Book reports pose a difficult challenge for students with VCFS because of their difficulty remembering and synthesizing the information they read. Devise a template and a strategy that these learners can use to read a novel or trade book. For example, the students might use a specially designed book to record relevant information as they read a chapter.

17. Expressive language is often an area of weakness for learners with VCFS. Many of these students will find it daunting to stand before their peers and present a project or report. How can a teacher help these students accomplish this skill? How can the classroom environment be altered to accommodate for a reluctant speaker?

18. Organizational skills continue to challenge many students with VCFS into adulthood. What are some ways that teachers can help students keep track of papers and due dates for assignments? How can parents work with the school to help insure the homework is completed and turned in on time? Do you think that students with VCFS should be held accountable for late work? Why or why not?

19. Discuss how you feel students with special needs should be graded in school. One student with VCFS in the United States was not voted into

the Honor Society by the school staff even though his grade point average was high enough to qualify and he had participated in the required community service projects. What do you think of this decision?

20. Many children with developmental delays will need to be taught life skills as they mature. For students who are mainstreamed into the regular education curriculum, this can pose a problem. How can the school incorporate this needed instruction in a program already filled with academic requirements? How would you arrange a program for a middle school student with VCFS that could address this issue?

21. In the United States, many students with VCFS graduate at age 18 even though they do not possess the skills they need for post-secondary education or for the workforce. Students with disabilities are entitled to be educated until age 21 by law. Research the transition programs that are available in your community. How could a higher functioning student with the VCFS learning profile be supported from age 19 to 21 in your area?

22. Part of any transition program for older students should include researching the available supports in the community for adults with disabilities. What are the adult programs available in your area? Do any of these programs require that the student remain in school until age 21 in order to receive services? What is the school's responsibility for arranging for the transfer of services from the school to the community agencies?

23. Students with special needs will need carefully orchestrated programs to help them plan for life as an adult. Design a program to assess the vocational options that might make a good match. Include both performance- and skill-based assessments in your program as well as opportunities for job shadowing and work experience.

24. Some students with VCFS have successfully attended a university or community college. What skills do you think a student must have to be able to make that transition? How is the special education program available at universities different from the services the student may have received in high school? Do students' rights differ? If so, how?

25. One huge challenge for students with VCFS is overcoming the lack of knowledge in both the educational and medical communities. How do you think the public can be made more aware of the syndrome? How can students with VCFS be taught to advocate for themselves?

# Index

## A

ABAS (Adaptive Behavior Assessment System), 30
Academic delay accommodations, 217-218
Accommodations. *See also educational level topics*
  for academic delay, 217-218
  for assignment organization, 218-219
  for behavior, 223-224
  of classroom environment, 221-222
  for evaluations, 219
  for fine visual/motor skill, 220-221
  for handwriting, 220-221
  home-school communication, 220
  for nonverbal learning disability (NVLD), 31-32, 224-226
  for notetaking, 222
  for organization, 218-219
  school-home communication, 220
  for testing, 219
  for test writing, 219-220
  for working memory, 222-223
Achenbach System of Empirically Based Assessment, 29
Adaptive Behavior Assessment System (ABAS), 30
ADD (attention deficit disorder), 132
ADHD (attention deficit hyperactivity disorder). *See also* Attention problems
  case study, 25, 61-62, 64-65
  cognitive remediation therapy, 162
  comorbidity, 43, 44
  and medication, 67
  neuroanatomy, 44
  as psychiatric issue, 60
ADI-R (Autism Diagnostic Interview-Revised), 30
ADOS (Autism Diagnostic Observation Schedule), 30
Adulthood transition (ages 18-21)
  case management, 209
  college, 211-212
  community support applications, 210-211
  difficulties of, 206-207
  finances, 207
  IDEA (Individuals with Disabilities Education Act), 211
  independent living skills, 210
  job interview skills, 209
  model program, 208-210
  outcomes expected, 207-208
  overview, 205
  postsecondary training, 211-212
  shared housing, 210
  Social Security benefits, 209, 210-211
  SSI (Supplemental Security Income), 211
  technical college, 209
  transition plan aspects, 207
  transition planning, 211
  tutoring, 208
  vocational rehabilitation, 210
  work experience, 209-210
Adult outcome longitudinal studies, 24-25
Albert Einstein College of Medicine, vii, 6

Anxiety disorders case study, 62–63
Arts classes, middle school, 188–189
ASD (atrial septal defect), 10
Assignment organization
        accommodations, 218–219
Attention deficit disorder (ADD), 132
Attention deficit hyperactivity disorder.
        *See* ADHD (attention deficit
        hyperactivity disorder)
Attention problems. *See also* ADHD
        (attention deficit hyperactivity
        disorder)
    and brain anatomy/physiology, 43–44
    overview, 22
    VCFS (velo-cardio-facial syndrome),
        41–44 (*See also* ADHD (attention
        deficit hyperactivity disorder)
Autism Diagnostic Interview-Revised
        (ADI-R ), 30
Autism Diagnostic Observation Schedule
        (ADOS), 30
Autism spectrum disorder, 23–24, 58, 153
Away-from-home experience, 189


**B**

Bal-A-Vix-X: Rhythmic, Balance/Auditory/
        Vision Exercises for Brain and
        Brain-Body Integration, 154
BASC (Behavior Assessment System for
        Children), 29
Bayley Scale, 17
Behavior. *See also under* Testing
    accommodations, 223–224
    case study, 232
    issue overview, 23–24
    Kindergarten–second grade (ages
        5-7), 154
    preschool intervention (ages 3–5),
        131–132
    stereotypic, 60
Behavior Assessment System for
        Children (BASC), 29
*The Berenstain Bears and the Messy
        Room* (Stan & Jan Berenstain),
        148
Bipolar disorder, 23
Birth to 3 intervention programs,
        117–118

Brain
    anatomy/physiology, 42, 44, 46, 49–51
    imaging studies, vii–viii, 40–41
Brain anatomy, 42, 44, 46
Brain Gym, 154
Bruininks-Orseretsky Test of Motor
        Proficiency, 21
Building Blocks software, 129


**C**

California Verbal Learning Test (CVLT),
        30
Camp Kodiak, 189
Case studies
    academic delay, 232
    ADHD (attention deficit hyperactivity
        disorder), 25, 61–62
    adolescents, 64–65
    adults, 25
    articulation difficulties, 230–231
    behavior problems, 232
    certificate of attendance diploma, 206
    depression, 25
    ear infection, 231
    expressive language skill deficits, 25
    high school student, 195–196
    hypertonia, 231
    independent living, 25
    Kindergarten–second grade (ages
        5-7), 155–156
    mathematics problems, 231–232
    OCD (obsessive-compulsive disorder),
        61–62, 64–65
    phobias, 61–62
    psychiatric issues, 61–63, 64–65
    schizo-affective disorder, 64–65
    school readiness, 231
    school services, 84, 85–93
    second grader, 155–156
    separation anxiety disorder, 64–65
    services qualification, 84, 85–93
    social skill deficits, 61–62
CBCL (Child Behavior Checklist), 29
CBM (curriculum-based measurement),
        114, 115
CBT (cognitive behavioral therapy), 65
CELF (Clinical Evaluation of Language
        Fundamentals), 30

CELF-P (Clinical Evaluation of Language Functions-Preschool), 78
CHARGE syndrome, 7
Child Behavior Checklist (CBCL), 29
Classroom environment accommodations, 221–222
Cleft palate
  case study, 62–63
  submucous, 10–11
  and VSD and subnormal IQ, 11
  and VSD (ventriculoseptal defect), 11
  without cleft lip, prevalence, 11
Clinical Evaluation of Language Functions-Preschool (CELF-P), 78
Clinical Evaluation of Language Fundamentals (CELF), 30
Cognition. *See also* IQ subnormalcy
  and academic performance, 39–40
  overview, 16–18
  testing caveats, 30–31
  and VSD and cleft palate, 11
Cognitive behavioral therapy (CBT ), 65
Cognitive remediation therapy, 162–163
Communication
  language skill, 77
  overview, 71–72
  speech, 72–77 (*See also main heading* Speech)
Comprehension overview, 22–23
Comprehensive Reading Assessment Battery, 167
Comprehensive Test of Phonological Processing (CTOPP), 145
Computers
  elementary grades 3–5 (ages 8–11), 163
  high school (ages 14–18), 186
  kindergarten–second grade (ages 5–7), 146–147, 149
  middle school (ages 11–14), 186
Connors Rating Scales-Revised (CRS-R), 29
Conotruncal anomalies face syndrome, 6. *See also* VCFS (velo-cardio-facial syndrome)
Continuous Performance Test-II (CPT), 29
CPT (Continuous Performance Test-II), 29

Curriculum based assessment (CBA ), 114, 115
Curriculum-based measurement (CBM), 114, 115
CVLT (California Verbal Learning Test), 30

**D**

DEC (Division for Early Childhood), Council for Exceptional Children, 123
del(7p) syndrome, 7
del(10p) syndrome, 7
Dennison, Paul, 154
Depakote, 67
Department of Education Institute of Education Sciences, 185–186
Depression, 25, 62
Diagnosis, viii, 12, 39–40
DIBELS (Dynamic Indicators of Basic Early Literacy Skills), 145
DiGeorge sequence, 7, 100
DiGeorge syndrome, 5, 7
Division for Early Childhood (DEC), Council for Exceptional Children, 123
Down, John Langon Haydon, 4
Down syndrome, viii, ix–xi, 4, 5, 7, 151
Dynamic Indicators of Basic Early Literacy Skills (DIBELS), 145
Dyscalculia, 128–130

**E**

Education. *See also* Intervention, educational
  and childhood illness, 95–102 (*See* Illness, childhood)
  language, 19–20
  learning issues, 25–28
  mathematics, 18–19, 45–47, 127–130, 149–152
    middle school (ages 11–14), 185–187
  NVLD (nonverbal learning disability), 31–32
  overview, 15
  planning for (*See* Cognition)

Education *(continued)*
  reading, 19
    elementary grades 3–5 (ages 8–11),
      166–169
    Kindergarten–second grade (ages
      5–7), 144–148
    middle school (ages 11–14),
      187–188
  VCFS intervention timeline, 32–34
  visual-spatial impairment, 18
Educational program planning, 230–235
Elementary grades 3–5 (ages 8–11). *See
    also main heading*
  Accommodations
  assignment recording, 162, 164
  cause/effect understanding, 167
  classroom environment, 170
  On Cloud Nine program, 171
  cognitive remediation therapy,
    162–163
  curriculum relevance, 161
  direct instruction, 170–171
  drill and practice, 161
  emotional issues, 174–175
  experiential approach, 172–173
  and fact/opinion, 167
  Fast ForWord program, 166
  file system, accordion, 164
  flash cards, 169, 170
  flexibility needs, 163–164
  friendship, 175
  gross motor activities, 174–175
  guided reading sheets, 161, 168
  hands-on approach, 172–173
  homework, 165–166
  Interact history simulations, 173
  involvement through activity, 161
  KWL (known, wants to know,
    learned) chart, 168, 169
  life skills, 175–176
  material abbreviation, 169
  mathematics, 170–172
  memorization, 170
  memory cues, 160–161
  Memory Matrix computer program,
    163
  mentors, community, 165–166
  music lessons, 175
  note provision, 161

  one-on-one settings, 160
  oral reading, 168
  organization skills, 163–165
  overview, 159–160
  prediction, 168
  projects, 169
  question answering, 169
  reading, 166–169
  reformatting reading text, 169
  remediation, 165–166
  reteaching process, 160–161
  schedule keeping, 162
  self-monitoring skill teaching, 169
  simulation approach, 173–174
  small group settings, 160, 169
  social issues, 174–175
  Structure of Intellect System, 162–163
  study guide provision, 161
  study skills, 163–165
  supplies organization, 165
  tape recorder use, 161, 168
  teasing, 175
  template provision, 162, 168, 169
  and test recall, 161
  text relevancy, 167
  The Thinker Math program, 171–172
  time organization, 165
  and tutors, 161, 165
  vocabulary of math, 171
  word banks, 161
  working memory deficits
    accommodations, 160–163,
      168–169
  written direction provision, 161
Executive function overview, 21–22
Expression variability, 9–10
Expressive One-Word Picture
    Vocabulary Test (EOWPVT), 78,
    88, 91

**F**

Fact sheet, 102–110
FAIS (Functional Assessment and
    Intervention System), 29
Fast ForWord program, 166, 187
Fetal alcohol syndrome, 5, 7
FISH (fluorescence in situ hybridization)
    screening, vii, 10

# BIBLIOGRAPHY/SUGGESTED READINGS

Allington, R. (2001). *What really matters for struggling readers.* Portsmouth, NH: Heinemann.

Annunziata, J., & Scott, M. (1998). *Help is on the way: A child's book about ADD.* Washington, DC: Magination Press.

Cain, B. S., & Patterson, A. (1990). *Double-dip feelings: Stories to help children understand emotions.* Washington, DC: Magination Press.

Catts, H. W., & Kamhi, A. G. (1999). *Language and reading disabilities.* Boston: Allyn and Bacon.

Curry, N. E., & Johnson, C. N. (1990). *Beyond self-esteem: Developing a genuine sense of human value.* Washington, DC: National Association for the Education of Young Children.

Elias, M. J., Friedlander, B. S., & Tobias, S. E. (2001). *Engaging the resistant child through computers: A manual to facilitate social and emotional learning.* Port Chester, NY: Dude.

Ferrara, J. M. (1996). *Peer mediation: Finding a way to care.* York, ME: Stenhouse.

Fountas, I. C., & Pinnell, G. S. (2001). *Guiding readers and writers grades 3–6, Teaching comprehension, genre, and content literacy.* Portsmouth, NH: Heinemann.

Gillet, J. W., & Temple, C. A. (1994). *Understanding reading problems: Assessment and instruction.* New York: HarperCollins College Publishers.

Gorman, J. C. (2001). *Emotional disorders & learning disabilities in the elementary classroom, Interactions and interventions.* Thousand Oaks, CA: Corwin Press.

Greenspan, S. I., Wieder, S., & Simons, R. (1998). *The child with special needs: Encouraging intellectual and emotional growth.* Reading, MA: Perseus Books.

Hallowell, E. M., & Ratey, J. J. (1995). *Driven to distraction, Recognizing and coping with attention deficit disorder from childhood through adulthood.* New York: Simon & Schuster.

Hallowell, E. M., & Ratey, J. J. (2005). *Delivered from distraction: Getting the most out of life with attention deficit disorder* (1st ed.). New York: Ballantine Books.

Hersen, M., & Rosqvist, J. (2005). *Encyclopedia of behavior modification and cognitive behavior therapy.* Thousand Oaks, CA: Sage.

Hong, E., & Milgram, R. M. (2000). *Homework: Motivation and learning preference.* Westport, CT: Bergin & Garvey.

Keefe, J. W., & Jenkins, J. M. (2000). *Personalized instruction: Changing classroom practice.* Larchmont, NY: Eye on Education.

Keene, E. O., & Zimmermann, S. (1997). *Mosaic of thought: Teaching comprehension in a reader's workshop.* Portsmouth, NH: Heinemann.

Koplow, L. (1991). *Tanya and the Tobo man: A story for children entering therapy.* New York: Magination Press.

Lavoie, R. D. (2005). *It's so much work to be your friend: Helping the child with learning disabilities find social success.* New York: Simon & Schuster.

Lazear, D. G., Ray, H., & Lazear, D. G. (1999). *Eight ways of knowing: Teaching for multiple intelligences: A handbook of techniques for expanding intelligence* (3rd ed.). Arlington Heights, IL: SkyLight Professional Development.

McConnell, K., & Ryser, G. (2005). *Practical ideas that really work for students with ADHD* (2nd ed.). Austin, TX: Pro-Ed.

McEwan, E. K. (2002). *Teach them all to read: Catching the kids who fall through the cracks*. Thousand Oaks, CA: Corwin Press.

McLaughlin, M., & Allen, M. (2002). *Guided comprehension: A teaching model for grades 3–8*. Newark, DE: International Reading Association.

Meyer, D. J. (1997). *Views from our shoes: Growing up with a brother or sister with special needs*. Bethesda, MD: Woodbine House.

Nadeau, K. G., & Dixon, E. B. (1997). *Learning to slow down and pay attention: A book for kids about ADD*. Washington, DC: Magination Press.

Naparstek, N. (2002). *Successful educators: A practical guide for understanding children's learning problems and mental health issues*. Westport, CT: Bergin & Garvey.

Olweus, D. (1993). *Bullying at school: What we know and what we can do*. Oxford: Cambridge.

Peterkin, A. (1992). *What about me? When brothers and sisters get sick*. New York: Magination Press.

Power, T. J., Karustis, J. L., & Habboushe, D. F. (2001). *Homework success for children with ADHD: A family-school intervention program*. New York: Guilford Press.

Quinn, P. O., & Stern, J. M. (1991). *Putting on the brakes: Young people's guide to understanding attention deficit hyperactivity disorder (ADHD)*. Washington, DC: Magination Press.

Rief, S. F. (2005). *How to reach and teach children with ADD/ADHD: Practical techniques, strategies, and interventions* (2nd ed.). San Francisco: Jossey-Bass.

Sarasin, L. C. (1998). *Learning style perspectives: Impact in the classroom*. Madison, WI: Atwood Pub.

Shapiro, A. H. (1999). *Everybody belongs: Changing negative attitudes toward classmates with disabilities*. New York: Garland.

Staub, D. (1998). *Delicate threads: Friendships between children with and without special needs in inclusive settings*. Bethesda, MD: Woodbine House.

Stern, J. M., & Ben-Ami, U. (1996). *Many ways to learn: Young people's guide to learning disabilities*. Washington, DC: Magination Press.

Tomlinson, C. A. (2003). *Fulfilling the promise of the differentiated classroom: Strategies and tools for responsive teaching*. Alexandria, VA: Association for Supervision and Curriculum Development.

Wetherby, A. M., & Prizant, B. M. (2000). *Autism spectrum disorders: A transactional developmental perspective*. Baltimore: P. H. Brookes.

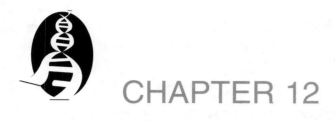

# CHAPTER 12

# Exploring New Horizons
## *Middle School (Ages 11–14)*

$A$s children mature and move on to middle school the issues involving students with VCFS become more complicated. Early adolescence is a time of turmoil and change in nearly all students. As they move from the nurturing elementary school atmosphere to the more demanding (and chaotic) middle school, they seek out acceptance from peers rather than adults. Students become much more concerned about what other students think about them and they worry about fitting in with crowd. Being "different" is usually not preferred and students will often go to great lengths to fit in.

For students with VCFS, reading social situations is difficult. They often don't see the humor in situations and may interpret remarks made by other students as teasing when that was not the intent. Poor communication skills can lead to difficulty offering back quick-witted comments or being able to converse about current topics of interest to others. This can negatively impact their ability to make and keep friends.

Finally, some children with VCFS have trouble with paying attention to personal hygiene. For example, they don't brush their teeth thoroughly or they may leave their hair uncombed. Sometimes they may have sloppy eating habits or may not realize their face needs cleaning. All of these situations can lead to embarrassment at school and rejection by peers.

Most children with VCFS are bright enough to realize whether or not they are popular and it makes a difference to them. Unlike students with more severe cognitive impairments, students with VCFS strive for acceptance. They want to succeed academically and socially. They want to be included in social events and a part of school life. Isolation and rejection can be a real problem at this age and steps should be taken to insure that the students with VCFS are comfortable at school and with peers.

## DRESS, GROOMING, AND HEALTH EDUCATION

Parents may need to take an active role in helping their child with VCFS look and act acceptable at school. This doesn't mean that families need to go out and purchase the latest fashions for their child. It may be worthwhile, however, for parents to observe how other children dress and then help their child select clothing to blend in. Years ago I taught a lovely young girl with a cognitive disability. Her mother dressed her in skirts with juvenile print patterns—typically worn by girls of a much younger age. The students at school were not overtly mean to this girl, but they didn't associate with her either. I felt her clothing was somewhat inappropriate for middle school and set her apart from others. After meeting with her parents and discussing the issue, she dressed differently. Toward the spring of the year she had made two new friends and became much happier at school.

Parents will also need to be directly involved with grooming needs and they should supervise these skills until the child is comfortable and competent on his or her own. Table manners should be taught and so should rules of etiquette. Students with VCFS can be taught to smile, greet others, and give compliments. They need to be taught tactful behavior and social graces. Do not assume children with VCFS will learn these skills on their own. Many of them do not generalize from observed behavior and they will need direct instruction. An excellent book entitled *What Does Everybody Else Know That I Don't? Social Skills Help for Adults with AD/HD* by Michele Novotni (Novotni & Peterson, 1999) can serve as a starting point for parents trying to teach these skills at home. There are also many books published for LD/ADD students that will help address this issue.

In addition, VCFS young adults will need direct instruction in the issues of human growth and development. Although many school districts offer sex education classes for middle school students, often these classes are part of a broader health curriculum and are not comprehensive. Parents and special education staff will need to individualize instruction to make sure the student understands the concepts presented.

Finally, parents of young teenagers may struggle with how to talk to their children about having velo-cardio-facial syndrome or whether to tell them at all. If the child asks questions about his or her medical situation, this would be a good time to begin this dialogue. Students at this age are old enough to understand basic genetic information and at some point they will need to be able to advocate for themselves. The Velo-Cardio-Facial Syndrome Educational

Foundation, http://www.vcsfef.org is a great source for current information about the syndrome. Trained counselors can also support young adults as they learn about their unique set of needs.

## LANGUAGE AND COMMUNICATION SKILLS

Intercommunication skills directly impact a student's ability to function effectively at school, at home, and in the community. Good communication skills:

- Allow people to develop positive relationships with others
- Facilitate coping successfully with the behavioral demands of specific settings
- Help individuals communicate their desires, wants, needs, and personal preferences
- Provide a foundation for competent performance in the academic, personal, vocational, and community arenas
- Allow a person to move freely within and throughout the community and to act appropriately in those settings

In order for students with VCFS to use language effectively as an adult, they will need to perfect three major skills:

1. Use language for different purposes (i.e., use appropriate tones or inflections for the situation)

2. Adapt their language to the listening audience or circumstance (use different language when addressing an adult as compared to a young child or know when it is appropriate to blurt out a comment)

3. Understand the rules for conversation (don't monopolize, take turns, listen, change topics tactfully, etc.)

It is not unusual for speech and language therapy to be needed throughout the middle and high school years. Therapists can help with social conversation skills, self-advocacy, academics, and understanding more complex language. In many schools, the speech and language specialist works right in the classroom to help children acquire these skills. Other districts use a pull-out or resource room model to deliver services. Parents may also consider investigating whether their health insurance covers private therapy. Sometimes additional help outside the school day is necessary to meet the higher academic demands of middle school. If additional help is possible it is best to coordinate services with the school so that therapy time is used wisely.

## ACADEMICS

There is a definite shift after fifth grade to a curriculum-driven model for academics. The emphasis of instruction changes from acquiring basic skills to applying learned skills to new subject areas. There is a much heavier emphasis on test taking as a means to measure academic progress and students are held more accountable for remembering subject matter. Students with VCFS will need additional supports to be able to succeed in a more intensely demanding environment. The following deficits often found in the VCFS population will need to be addressed in the middle school child's educational plan.

### Working Memory Impairment

Working memory impairment may be the most problematic deficit for a VCFS student to overcome. Many children with VCFS cannot store more than one or two pieces of information in memory at one time. For example, if they are asked to compare/contrast the characters in two books, they will have difficulty thinking about the first character while they are trying to remember attributes of the second character. Or in a class discussion, it will be hard to remember the thread of the conversation to comment on a previous point made by a student. They will not be able to recall a complex set of directions or remember the details of an assignment. One parent described her child as seemingly going along in a fog. Her son attended class regularly, but could not explain what occurred during the day with any detail or retell the requirements of an assignment. He often could remember bits and pieces of discussions, but would mix up important facts or would totally miss the point of the lesson. His mom would get frustrated trying to help him finish assignments at home because she did not have a clear understanding of the teacher's expectations. Her son could not understand why school was so confusing and felt that he was working hard to succeed, but he was "stupid." It is easy to see how this situation could spiral into a downward path of self-doubt and low self-esteem.

Accommodations for working memory deficits are listed in Chapter 11 and Appendix A. Most importantly at this age level, teachers must understand the problem and realize that it is imperative for the student with VCFS to have a written copy of all class notes and assignment expectations. Sometimes one student in class can use carbonless paper to make a set of notes for the student, but this will work better at the high school or college level. At middle school, notes may have to be provided by an educational assistant, adult volunteer, regular education teacher, or learning disabilities specialist. The teacher should provide a detailed explanation of projects and assignments that explains all of the aspects of the requirements. Many teachers do this already for all their students. However, because of the working memory issues with VCFS, this should be addressed in the VCFS student's IEP. A step-by-step listing of expectations, due dates, and relevant information in written form will allow the student to reread the directions multiple times and refer to the list as he or she is completing the assignment.

In addition, templates that help a child retain necessary information for further use can be helpful. For example, since many students with VCFS struggle quite a bit with mathematics, more complex problems will present a challenge. This is especially true with multistep problem-solving tasks. A template could be used that would direct the students to record relevant information as they work through a problem.

Example:

Suppose a person bought three shirts for $28.00 each and paid 5% sales tax. What would be the final cost of the purchase?

Template:

Find and write the cost of the shirts _____

Find and write the amount of sales tax _____

Find the total cost _____

Notice this template did not tell the student what operation to do to find the cost of the shirts, nor did it instruct the student how to find sales tax or the total amount. The goal would be for the student to be able to apply understanding of math to do these steps independently. It does, however, instruct students to write down the answers they got to the smaller steps of the problem so that they can use these answers to solve the larger total cost question. These templates can be color coded, enlarged, and reproduced to make the working memory impairment less problematic for the student. They can be tailored to meet the needs of students as they gain more confidence and expertise in their skills. Other accommodations that are helpful include word banks, open book tests, notes for tests, recording of ideas, guided reading sheets, and fill-in-the-blank story maps (see Appendix A).

### *Training in Memory Techniques and Cognitive Remediation Therapy*

Mnemonic devices are specific ways to help people remember and recall information. Mnemonic techniques can be used effectively to mentally retrieve facts for a test or to help make associations between two or more units of information. There is quite a bit of research supporting the use of memory strategies with learning disabled students (Levin, 1993; R. Brigham & M. Brigham, 2001).

Mnemonic strategies rely on both words and imagery to help recall information. According to M. A. Mastropieri and T. E. Scruggs (1991), some of the more useful strategies are as follows:

■ First letter mnemonics, acronyms, and acrostics: First letter mnemonics or acronyms use the first letter of each word or phrase to be recalled to form a meaningful word or phrase. For example, the word "homes" can help recall the names of the Great Lakes: Huron, Ontario, Michigan, Erie, and Superior. Acrostics support memory by creating an entire sentence to help recall information. In math, the order of operations for solving calculations (parentheses, exponents, multiplication, division, addition, and subtraction) can be remembered by using the phrase, "**P**lease **e**xcuse **m**y **d**ear **A**unt **S**ally."

■ Peg words: This strategy is helpful if the order of information to be recalled is important or when the information to be remembered is numerical. For example, suppose a student needed to remember five reasons in decreasing order of plausibility for the extinction of the dinosaurs. First the numbers one to five are each associated with a peg word. One = sun, two = shoe, three = tree, four = door, five = dive. If the first reason is the theory that a meteor hit the earth, the student could visualize a dinosaur in a field with a meteor flying past the sun. Later when the student thought of the first reason, he or she could recall one, then sun, then the meteor picture to remember the first fact. Locations can also be used as pegs to remember information. Students can visualize walking into school (one), passing the office (two), etc. Information to be recalled can be visualized in relationship to the location. As a dinosaur entered the school it got hit in the head with a meteor. When it progressed to the drinking fountain there was no water (reason number two for dinosaur extinction was the swamps dried up).

■ Keywords: The keyword strategy uses three steps. First, reconstruct the term to be remembered into a word that is similar in sound, already familiar, and easily pictured. Second, relate the keyword to the term to be learned with a fun picture or image. Finally, retrieve the appropriate term by mentally visualizing the keyword, picture, and what was happening in the picture. For example, if a student needed to remember that the capital of Kentucky was Frankfort, he or she could visualize a boy standing in the middle of the state of Kentucky munching on a frankfurter. Or if the student needed to recall Springfield is the capital of Illinois, he or she could picture springing (or actually physically spring) off a chair while shouting, "Illinois." Keywords have been shown to be an effective technique across a wide range of subject areas (Swanson, 1999; Scruggs & Mastropieri, 1992).

Although these techniques can be used successfully with younger students, middle school may be a more appropriate age to try to teach these tools to students with VCFS. Even with formal instruction in the devices, it may be necessary for a tutor, parent, or teacher to help the student determine how to use the techniques in a particular situation. The tutor may ask the student, "How are you going to remember this information?" Then time can be spent helping the student think of keywords or perhaps an acrostic to apply to the specific material to be studied. The adult should try to relate the keyword or saying to something meaningful to the student (like the name of a favorite pet). Do not expect the student with VCFS to be readily able to apply these memory tricks without assistance. It is reasonable, however, to believe that if a memory tool is decided upon and used with drill and practice, it will help in memory recall.

## Visual Perceptual Impairments

A second area of impairment that causes difficulty for middle school students with this syndrome is visual perceptual deficits. Adults with VCFS consistently do poorly on tests of visual memory and visual form constancy. Visual form constancy is the ability to recognize original shapes in a rotated position or to find a shape hidden in an environment. How this impairment affects learning is still being studied. However, it may impact a student's ability to locate objects in a cluttered environment (such as a school locker) or to recognize different fonts or text. They may also have difficulty in mathematics when they are asked to rotate shapes in space in isometric problems or to apply measurement formulas to geometric shapes. Accommodations for visual perceptual deficits can include enlarging print, reducing unnecessary print on a page, labeling containers for locker storage, using a color-coded accordion folder for storing papers, and allowing extra time for finding misplaced items (see Appendix A). Occupational therapists should assess all students with VCFS for these deficits and if necessary they can provide specific therapy to target this area.

## Mathematics

Students will need to continue with the programs from elementary school and the after-school assistance to help address their math needs (see Chapters 10 and 11) Careful assessment of math competencies will help identify areas of weakness so appropriate remedial measures can be taken. Care should be taken to be realistic about the amount of work assigned so that students are not overwhelmed. The What Works Clearinghouse (http://www.what works.ed.gov) was " . . . established in 2002 by the U.S. Department of Education's Institute of Education Sciences to provide educators, policymakers, researchers, and the public with a central and trusted source of scientific evidence of what works in education." The topic of middle school mathematics was one of the first areas addressed by this group. Several math programs have been assessed for their effectiveness, but there are a limited number of studies that have passed the What Works Panel for reliable scientific evidence. In addition, the studies did not specifically look at how the programs improved outcomes for special education students.

Nevertheless, two math programs, the I CAN Learn Mathematics Curriculum and the Cognitive Tutor, did show statistically significant improvement in students' math skills. The Interactive Computer-Aided Natural Learning (I CAN Learn®) program is an education software system that delivers algebra and pre-algebra courses to middle and high school students. The I CAN Learn curriculum is designed for students to work at their own pace in a classroom with a one-to-one ratio of students to computers. Each interactive lesson uses the direct instruction method and includes a pretest, review, lesson presentation, guided practice, and posttest. Also included are cumulative reviews, real-world applications, and cumulative tests to determine retention. According to the publishers, the I CAN Learn curriculum incorporates national and state performance standards, and can be configured to meet state and local Grade Level Expectations (GLEs). Carnegie Learning is the company that produces the Cognitive Tutor program. This program also uses the computer as a component in its program and accompanies it with teacher-led activities, drill and practice, and textbook exercises.

The direct instruction, computer-based platform of the I CAN Learn program seems like a good fit for students with VCFS. However, it would be necessary to have a special education teacher or aide working alongside students with VCFS to make sure they are making the connections needed as they progress through a computer program. Many students with VCFS do not problem-solve well independently, so they will need assistance understanding the computer-generated concepts. Given this additional support, this program as well as the Cognitive Tutor curriculum may be a good choice.

For drill with basic computation, students might enjoy doing sheets like those in the program *Middle School Math with Pizzazz* (1989) by Steve and Janis Marcy. This program uses puzzles and jokes to make the math practice more fun. Students are asked a riddle at the top of each page like, "What do they call cows in Alaska? or "What happened when Count Dracula met a pretty girl?" After correctly doing a set of math problems they are able to decode the answers—(e.g., "Eskimoos," or "It was love at first bite"). These sheets are highly motivating and provide the student with immediate feedback as to whether their answers are right. These books can be purchased on-line at http://www.wrightgroup.com or through Creative Publications.

Many students with VCFS can learn more difficult math concepts, including algebra, if the skills are taught in a step-by-step fashion. When the math involves a lot of writing, such as happens with a more involved algebra problem, some students with VCFS will need additional support to avoid mistakes.

It might be helpful to have an aide or other adult assist the student with writing and recording the information. It might be helpful to do the work on a chalkboard or on graph paper. Remember the issues with the working memory and try to assist the student with recording all steps of the problem. Even though the student may know what to do, he or she may not be able to carry out all steps of the problem without a careless error. It may be necessary to offer this added assistance and also to give partial credit for problems correctly attempted. The key here is for teachers to be flexible with grading and to understand the memory/attention issues associated with the syndrome. A teacher who only rewards completely correct answers may not be the best match for a student with VCFS.

## Reading Instruction

Reading instruction at middle school focuses on higher level thinking skills and comprehension. Students with VCFS often have difficulty with both of these areas. Relatively strong decoding skills mask the fact that the student really does not understand the nuances of the story or novel. The suggestions for assisting with reading at the upper elementary school level (see Chapter 11) will also be helpful at this level. Additionally, there are some other possibilities for remediation.

The Read 180 program, A Comprehensive Reading Intervention Solution, is a program that targets adolescent illiteracy using technology, print, and professional development. It can be accessed at http://www.teacher.scholastic.com. Students use adaptive software and high interest literature and receive direct instruction to improve reading, writing, and vocabulary skills. This program is intensive and students must use the materials for several hours a day. The research on this program from field studies is promising. It seems to be a good fit for students with VCFS because it heavily relies on computers and direct instruction. Some schools use this program as a substitute for the regular English class typically taught at middle school.

Fast ForWord, at http://www.scilearn.com, also has a program specifically tailored for older students. It uses age-appropriate graphics and contexts to build fundamental cognitive skills in the areas of memory, attention, processing, and sequencing. The series moves on with Fast ForWord Language to Reading and a Fast ForWord Reading Series. The Kumon reading program, at http://www.Kumon.com, also has middle school appropriate levels and can be used to supplement the reading instruction provided by the school.

As with math, the key for success at this level is creativity and flexibility on the part of the teacher. Students will need assistance reading full-length novels, especially those typically taught at this level. Preteaching that foreshadows action in the story, vocabulary building, and background scene setting are all helpful strategies to assist with comprehension. Students with VCFS should meet one-on-one or in a small group with an aide or teacher to verbally check for understanding. They should be encouraged to write down or word process key information as they are reading. Study guides and guided reading sheets should also be used to help students retain important story information.

## Social Studies and Science

Success in the social studies and science areas is highly dependent on the accommodations that can be offered. Students with VCFS will have difficulty in a social studies class that has a lecture delivery model with tests. Unfortunately, this approach to instruction is too often used in middle level classes. Even in classes with small group discussions, it is often extremely difficult for the VCFS student to follow the conversation and learn. Reading a textbook and comprehending the information will also prove problematic without additional support. The suggestions for simulation activities mentioned in Chapter 11 will work well both at this level and at high school.

In science, especially in a lab setting, it will be hard for the student to understand the concept demonstrated without direct assistance and further examples. Students with VCFS who are mainstreamed into regular education classes may need the support of an aide, tutor, or special education resource teacher to help reteach the concepts taught in a large group format. Additional time devoted to restate the concepts in simpler language would help solidify the content.

Teachers will need to furnish the student with study guides and notes from class. It may also be necessary to modify tests and/or perhaps allow the student opportunities to demonstrate knowledge through a project or paper. Students would also benefit from test retake opportunities.

Teachers can also access Appendix A to see the lists of accommodations that might help students be successful in their classes.

## Related Arts Classes and Foreign Language Instruction

Many times it is easy to overlook the need to educate related arts teachers about the unique needs of special education students. It is imperative, however, that all teachers working with students with VCFS understand the syndrome and program accordingly. The physical education, art, music, and consumer education teachers all need to realize the need to repeat directions, offer written instructions, supply notes, and give additional help. Each class will have its own set of challenges. The gym teacher, for example, will need to know about the organization trouble, hearing difficulties in a large gym, and perhaps the need for additional assistance with the combination lock. The art teacher may need information about fine motor coordination and visual/spatial issues. In reality, middle school students may have as many as eight different teachers during the course of a day. The syndrome-related difficulties follow the student from class to class, regardless of course content. Failing a related arts class can be as devastating to a student's self-esteem as a poor grade in an academic area.

One area that should be given serious consideration and additional attention is music. If possible, willing students with VCFS should be given an opportunity to participate in band, orchestra, or some type of instrument instruction. It is unclear why this occurs, but many children with this syndrome seem to excel in music. Several have pursued music careers and others have found friendships through their music involvement. A flexible approach to teaching music may be necessary to find an approach that works well with a given student. However, this is a class that may offer a positive outlet in a demanding academic day.

## AWAY FROM HOME EXPERIENCE

This age is a good time to consider arranging for an away from home experience for a child with VCFS. Many typically developing children at this age level enjoy going to summer camp for several weeks in between academic terms. However, finding a suitable camping experience can be difficult for children with chronic health/developmental issues. Many children with VCFS would have difficulty attending a typical camp because they would need their medication/health needs monitored and they may find the stress of being away from home difficult to handle. Many higher functioning preteens with VCFS also would not fit in at a camp for more severely impaired teens, especially if they have been educated in a regular classroom environment.

One option to consider is a camp such as the Victory Junction Camp in Randleman, North Carolina. This camp is a member of the Hole-in-the-Wall Gang Camps, which provide children with chronic and life-threatening illness an opportunity to participate in a camping experience. In 2005, this camp began to accept campers with genetic disorders for a specialized neurology/genetics summer camp week. Several children with VCFS attended this camp and had a successful and memorable experience (Goldenberg, 2006). The camp is free of charge.

A second option is Camp Kodiak north of Toronto in Canada. This is a noncompetitive special needs camp for children with learning difficulties and/or ADD. The camp has a small camper-to-staff ratio and has trained medical staff available at all times. This camp has also provided successful camping experiences for children and young adults with VCFS, so the staff is familiar with the syndrome. There is also an opportunity for a counselor in training program for older VCFS teens. Additional information on Camp Kodiak can be found at http://www.campkodiak.com.

## REFERENCES

Brigham. F. J., & Brigham, M. M. (1998). Using keyword mnemonics in general music classes. Cognitive psychology meets music history. *Journal of Research and Development in Education, 31*(4), 205–213.

Brigham, R., & Brigham, M. (2001). A focus on mnemonic instruction. Current Practice Alerts, *Division for Learning Disabilities and Division for Research of the Council of Exceptional Children, 5*. Retrieved 2006 from http://www.dldcec.org/alerts/

Goldenberg, P. (2006). *Summer camping experience with children and adolescents with 22q11.2 deletion at Victory Junction in Randleman, North Carolina.* Poster presentation at the12th Annual Scientific Meeting, Strasbourg, France.

Levin, J. R. (1993). Mnemonic strategies and classroom learning: A twenty-year report card. *The Elementary School Journal, 94* (2), 235–244.

Marcy, S., & Marcy, J. (1989). *Middle school math with pizzazz.* Mountain View, CA: Creative Publications.

Mastropieri, M. A., & Scruggs, T. E. (1991). *Teaching students ways to remember: Strategies for learning mnemonically.* Cambridge, MA: Brookline Press.

Novotni, M., & Peterson, R. (1999). *What does everybody else know that I don't? Social skills help for adults with AD/HD.* North Branch, MN: Specialty Press.

Scruggs, T. E., & Mastropieri, M. A. (1992). Classroom application of mnemonic instruction: Acquisition, maintenance, and generalization. *Exceptional Children, 58,* 219–229.

Swanson, H. L. (1999). *Interventions for students with learning disabilities. A meta-analysis of treatment outcomes.* New York: Guilford Press.

The What Works Clearinghouse. (2006). Retrieved May, 2006, from http://www.what works.ed.gov

## BIBLIOGRAPHY/SUGGESTED READINGS

Allen, J. (1995). *It's never too late: Leading adolescents to lifelong literacy.* Portsmouth, NH: Heinemann.

Barkley, R. A. (2000). *Taking charge of ADHD: The complete, authoritative guide for parents.* New York: Guilford Press.

Barkley, R. A., & Benton, C. M. (1998). *Your defiant child: 8 steps to better behavior.* New York: Guilford Press.

Blotzer, M. A., & Ruth, R. (1995). *Sometimes you just want to feel like a human being: Case studies of empowering psychotherapy with people with disabilities.* Baltimore: P. H. Brookes.

Bogdan, R., & Taylor, S. J. (1994). *The social meaning of mental retardation: Two life stories.* New York: Teachers College Press.

Brolin, D. E. (1995). *Career education: A functional life skills approach.* Englewood Cliffs, NJ: Merrill.

Chazan, M. (1998). *Helping socially withdrawn and isolated children and adolescents.* London: Cassell.

Clough, P. (2005). *Handbook of emotional & behavioural difficulties.* London: Sage.

Deshler, D. D., Ellis, E. S., & Lenz, B. K. (1996). *Teaching adolescents with learning disabilities: Strategies and methods.* Denver: Love Publishing.

Howley, M., & Arnold, E. (2005). *Revealing the hidden social code: Social stories for people with autistic spectrum disorders.* London: J. Kingsley.

Juvonen, J., & Graham, S. (2001). *Peer harassment in school: The plight of the vulnerable and victimized.* New York: Guilford Press.

Katz, N. H., & Lawyer, J. W. (1993). *Conflict resolution: Building bridges.* Thousand Oaks, CA: Corwin Press.

Katz, N. H., & Lawyer, J. W. (1994). *Preventing and managing conflict in schools.* Thousand Oaks, CA: Corwin Press.

Katz, N. H., & Lawyer, J. W. (1994). *Resolving conflict successfully: Needed knowledge and skills.* Thousand Oaks, CA: Corwin Press.

Kavale, K. A., & Mostert, M. P. (2004). *The positive side of special education: Minimizing its fads, fancies, and follies.* Lanham, MD: ScarecrowEducation.

King, G. A., Brown, E. G., & Smith, L. K. (2003). *Resilience: Learning from people with disabilities and the turning points in their lives.* Westport, CT: Praeger.

McCord, J. (1995). *Coercion and punishment in long-term perspectives.* New York: Cambridge University Press.

Minskoff, E. H., & Allsopp, D. (2003). *Academic success strategies for adolescents with learning disabilities and ADD.* Baltimore: P. H. Brookes.

Quinn, P. O. (1995). *Adolescents and ADD: Gaining the advantage.* New York: Magination Press.

Rathvon, N. (1999). *Effective school interventions: Strategies for enhancing academic achievement and social competence.* New York: Guilford Press.

Seligman, M. (1995). *The optimistic child: A revolutionary program that safeguards children against depression & builds lifelong resilience.* New York: Houghton Mifflin.

Thacker, J., Strudwick, D., & Babbedge, E. (2002). *Educating children with emotional and behavioural difficulties: Inclusive practice in mainstream schools.* London: Routledge/Falmer.

Tomlinson, C. A., & Eidson, C. C. (2003). *Differentiation in practice: A resource guide for differentiating curriculum, grades 5–9.* Alexandria, VA: Association for Supervision and Curriculum Development.

Waterman, J., & Walker, E. (2001). *Helping at-risk students: A group counseling approach for grades 6–9.* New York: Guilford Press.

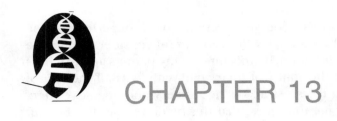

## CHAPTER 13

# Choices and Future Goals

## *High School (Ages 14–18)*

*P*oem by VCFS young adult entering high school:

At first . . .

I was nervous

I was scared

I didn't know anyone

I was told everyone was nice and accepting here

I was told I would do fine.

It began . . .

People were all around

Insults were flying left and right

I felt alone and unwanted

I didn't know where to go or what to do

It grew worse and worse.

But then . . .

I became more outgoing.

I was fun to be around.

I taught myself to have fun.

I became happier.

More excited to be here.

This made me realize who I am

High school options, appropriate course selections, work experiences, college, and adult life—all of these topics will need careful consideration as the child with VCFS moves to adulthood. By this time, many parents and teachers have a fairly realistic idea of the ability of their child with VCFS. If the school has not done recent testing to assess academic mastery and cognitive functioning, this would be the time to request that this be done. It is also helpful to look outside of the school setting to the services of a neuropsychologist or psychiatrist. Several areas should be targeted including memory, processing speed, expressive/receptive language skills, academic skills (math, reading, written language), problem-solving ability, life skills, visual/auditory processing, and vocational aptitude. These results, as well as a careful look at the student's school functioning, will help the educational planning team make sound decisions regarding an appropriate high school program. *It should be stressed, again, that there is a wide range of variability associated with this syndrome.* Some less affected students have successfully graduated from college with degrees and have gone on to hold professional jobs. For them, a college prep curriculum was the appropriate route to take. For others, a work focus/technical school model was a better choice. In either case, all students with VCFS should work toward achieving a regular high school diploma. It is vitally important that a great deal of information is gathered and time is spent discussing/exploring the various options available. The vast majority of students with VCFS will be able to do some type of work (full- or part-time) as adults. No parent wants to see an adult child sitting home with no purpose to the day and no job possibilities. The trick is to find an area of interest that is a realistic goal and move forward in a systematic fashion to achieve it.

## COLLEGE PREP CONSIDERATION

If the student with VCFS has been reasonably successful at managing the academic demands of school up until this point, a college prep curriculum should be carefully considered. With the tutoring and the academic supports provided by many colleges and universities, the disabled student has many opportunities available. All campuses have centers that specialize in providing accommodations to students. High school students should take all of the coursework necessary for admission to college. The high school guidance department will have literature on what the requirements are and can advise students how to plan their high school years to prepare for the demands of college coursework. Students should inquire about the foreign language requirement for admission to the schools they are interested in attending. *Many universities waive this requirement for students who have documented language disabilities.* Students are sometimes allowed to substitute other coursework (like signing for the hearing impaired) instead of struggling through learning a foreign language.

## PUBLIC VERSUS PRIVATE HIGH SCHOOL OPTIONS

Some students with VCFS who found it difficult to manage in a regular public school have chosen instead to attend a college prep program in a school that specializes in learning disabilities. These schools have smaller student-to-teacher ratios and may help prepare students for independent living and college life. The drawback of these programs, especially the overnight ones, is the expense, which can be as high as $30,000 per year and more. In addition, parents are at a greater distance from their child and may not have good insight into problems (especially in the social/emotional area) that can arise. Nevertheless, there are some success stories from private school attendance. This is certainly an option worth exploring. There are several Web sites with private school information online. Parents are strongly encouraged to contact the schools personally and disclose information about their child and VCFS. It is imperative that a student's situation is known so that the school can assess whether its program would be a good match.

## TECHNICAL SCHOOL OPTIONS

Public high schools can be large, daunting places for all new incoming students. High schools are usually larger, less personal, and more rigid than middle schools. The focus shifts from student centered to curriculum centered where mastery of content is the driving force. Many campuses are competitive and college prep focused where technical training is discouraged and choice is limited to what sections of biology are available rather than what other science courses might be an option. Some schools give little attention to alternative class options and pressure is on the students to pass high-stakes tests to graduate. Students with disabilities can become overwhelmed with this type of setup and many drop out or end up receiving a certificate of attendance rather than a regular diploma. A well-written IEP is the first step in tailoring the school environment to better fit the needs of the child with VCFS. Even a carefully crafted IEP, however, will not totally revamp the focus of the high school. It might be necessary to "think out of the box" and carefully explore all the possibilities for secondary school available in a given geographical area. Perhaps a magnet school with a music emphasis would be a good alternative, or maybe the technical school in the other part of town.

## CASE VIGNETTE

John was a 15-year-old student with VCFS when he entered high school in an upper middle class suburban city in the United States. The high school, a nationally recognized school of excellence, prided itself on the number of national merit scholars it produced and the long record of success in athletic competitions. It had a rigorous curriculum and high expectations for its students. The staff had never heard of velo-cardio-facial syndrome.

John had worked hard in middle school, earned good grades with support from special education teachers, played in the school band, and had a few friends. He had a full scale IQ of 87 and expressive language difficulties that interfered with friendships, and he struggled academically—especially with test taking, reading comprehension, and math. He often complained about teasing from peers and worried about fitting in with others. Nonetheless, he was relatively successful at school with special education support.

The first year of high school proved to be particularly difficult. The academic demands of the classes became much more rigorous and teachers were reluctant to allow accommodations. They were more punitive regarding issues like late work or misinterpretation of directions. The school was large and impersonal. Students in "remedial" classes often exhibited belligerent behavior, had truancy issues, and were involved with gangs. John was the target of threats, vandalism, and taunting.

As the year progressed, the problems began spinning out of control. John had outbursts of anger at home which shifted from rage to threat of suicide. In an effort to make school less stressful, John's parents met frequently with staff to try to advocate for better understanding of the VCFS challenges, more services for tutoring, and better monitoring of friendship/peer issues. They also inquired about the school's vocational options other than a four-year college prep curriculum.

The meetings were not productive and the staff struggled to come up with a suitable program. The situation became increasingly tense. John sought psychological help and was placed on medication for mood swings and anxiety. Finally toward spring, the decision was made to seek a change in placement. John's parents sold their home and moved to a nearby school district where the high school offered a wider range of classes for differing ability levels and the school's climate was more positive. The problems were not totally eliminated, but the change presented a new perspective, more positive role models, and an opportunity to deal with a different special education staff. John subsequently graduated from this high school, successfully attended a community college, works part-time, and is psychologically stable.

One place to go for help in deciding on a career and high school program would be to a person or agency that specializes in vocational training. Vocational rehabilitation experts can give advice on possible jobs for persons with disabilities. They have tests and questionnaires that look at a client's ability to learn new information, manipulate tools, focus on a job task, complete work within a time period, etc. They also can narrow down a person's interests into job possibilities. This added information can help assess the technical skills a person would need for a job and the high school program chosen in order to give opportunities to the student in these areas.

Students with VCFS often learn best in a program that is experiential in nature. This hands-on approach creates an environment where students can master skills in steps and then apply theory within a real life context. Technical schools that offer opportunities for job skill training might be a good alternative for students who struggle in a competitive academic environment.

Job experience courses are great ways for students to experiment with a specific job choice. Students earn high school credit and, in some cases, a salary for working at a job. A teacher is assigned to monitor job performance and to help the student develop successful job habits. The staff member also serves as a liaison between the employer and the student. This can help the student better understand the expectations of the employer and hopefully gain insight into the world of work. Students might attend the high school for a portion of the day and then leave campus to go to a job. This job experience can later be used to enhance a resume and to pave the way to employment once the student graduates. Many high schools have this type of program available to students. The IEP team can determine if this would be an option to consider.

## ACADEMICS

As stated earlier, the academics at the high school level are curriculum driven with emphasis on mastering content. Regardless of the subject, high school level courses are rigorous and challenging and demand higher level thinking skills. All students need to attend class regularly, hand in work on time, study seriously for tests, organize their work, and actively participate in class activities. They must be able to synthesize information, make inferences, respond critically, and successfully complete long-term projects. These skills demand a good memory, planning ability (executive functioning), organizational strategies, and the ability to think abstractly. Many students with VCFS have deficits in all of these areas and they will need daily assistance and monitoring to be successful.

There are numerous accommodations that the high school can provide to make the rigors of high school manageable. Many of these are listed in Appendix A at the end of the book. A few, however, are so important they are mentioned here.

First and foremost, all students with VCFS need a staff member who is available daily to help with organizational tasks. This person should be in frequent communication with the student's teachers to validate assignment expectations and due dates. A planner/calendar is essential to determine a daily schedule for task completion and a strategy for managing long-term projects. Since many students with VCFS have difficulty with transition, it would be helpful if this staff member was available before the beginning of the school year to help the student acclimate to a new environment. Perceptual difficulties may make navigating a new school or understanding a new schedule daunting. A friendly staff member can ease fears and provide additional assistance.

Second, scaffolding (allowing the student to obtain additional support while learning a new skill) will be needed across all curricular areas. This can be administered via a tutor, by a teacher aide, or through special education resources. The staff member should present the information in a very organized, systematic, and linear fashion. As the student becomes more proficient, he or she can move on to working independently on the material. Schools should not rely on peer tutors to provide this specialized instruction.

It is also important to reteach important concepts and whenever possible to relate the idea to a concrete situation the student has experienced. Many students with VCFS rely on rote strategies for remembering information, so their knowledge can be isolated, disconnected, and inefficiently accessed. They will need intervention to connect a current lesson to a topic that they have studied in the past. For example, if the student currently is working, relating a historical event (like a union strike) to the student's job would help make the abstract concept more relevant. Videos can also be used to help bring classroom subjects to life. If possible, field trips to places of interest (like the capitol or a museum) can also help. One point should be mentioned, however. A student with VCFS usually does not understand information presented in a large group format. Guided museum tours or large group lectures are not the preferred mode of instruction. Rather, use one-on-one or small group presentations, along with frequent comprehension checks, to teach material.

Third, all students with VCFS should be given preferential seating in the classroom and provided with handouts, notes, and study guides. Strategies for memorizing material and mastering content will have to be taught to the student with VCFS. A study guide provided before a test is helpful for condensing information and could be written into the educational plan. Studying should be divided into small chunks over several days to help the student commit the information into memory. Remember, the student with VCFS will need many more repetitions to remember information than the average student.

Fourth, it is also necessary to provide direct instruction and not to expect students with VCFS to discover theorems or concepts by doing classroom activities. These students will likely have particular difficulty applying problem-solving techniques in situations where models of solutions are not available or when they have to take responsibility for generating their own problem-solving strategies. This discovery learning approach has been popular with many math and science teachers in recent years. While this method might have advantages for normally developing students, this educational model is not recommended for students with VCFS. These students do not readily make connections between ideas, problem solve easily, or apply learned information to new ideas. Their organizational difficulties may lead to insecurity and they may tend to withdraw or shut down. This deficit is hard to overcome and it is a large aspect of their disability. Instead, they learn best by direct instruction, modeling, and hands-on learning. An approach that requires the student to actively participate in learning by practicing skills works better. One study that utilized computers to help with instruction showed positive results with a VCFS population (Kok & Soloman, 1995). A computer approach, therefore, might be helpful with teaching reading comprehension or math concepts.

Fifth, allow students to word process all written work and provide specific templates, instructions, and requirements for all assignments. This will assist both the student with VCFS and the adult tutor providing the scaffolding instruction. Try to eliminate the use of verbal multitask directions that will likely not be remembered completely or correctly.

Finally, high school teachers of students with VCFS will need to be understanding and flexible. One quality possessed by many students with this syndrome is their desire to please others and their willingness to try their best. Rigid teachers, who do not take time to understand this disability, may not appreciate the frustration that accompanies repeated failures and struggles to learn. Educators who allow these students to retake exams, do alternative projects, have additional time to complete assignments, hand in forgotten overdue work, and perhaps do extra credit are a better instructional match.

See Appendix A for lists of other academic accommodations to consider.

## OTHER CONSIDERATIONS FOR HIGH SCHOOL STUDENTS

### Driving Instruction

The decision to train young adults with VCFS to drive is a difficult one and should be carefully considered. Of paramount concern is whether or not they will be able to operate a vehicle safely. Will they be able to respond quickly to driving hazards? Will they fully understand the rules of the road? Will they use good judgment in inclement weather? The answers to these questions depends on the individual teenager. Many young adults with this syndrome do drive and are able to safely operate their vehicle. Learning to drive requires active participation and this mode of instruction works well for most individuals with VCFS. If they are given multiple opportunities for practice, one-on-one instruction on the rules of the road, and perhaps an extended drivers training class, many can be successful.

Driving is important. It supports a person's ability to be an independently functioning adult. It allows more job possibilities, increases options for social interactions, and improves one's access to the community. Depending on the living environment, driving can have a tremendous impact on quality of life. The decision to try to teach a teenager with disabilities to drive, however, must be weighed against the risk that the task is too complex. Parents of teenagers with VCFS should consult with others including the driver's education teachers, counselors, and special education instructors to get feedback as to whether their child would be able to master driving skills.

If teenagers with VCFS do pursue a driving license they may need some additional assistance in the areas of map reading, following directions, understanding what they need to do in case of an accident, and maintaining their vehicle. One accommodation that is very helpful is a computerized navigation system (GPS). These systems are available built into newer cars or they can be purchased separately to mount onto older models. Once an address is typed into the system, a voice guides the driver to the desired destination. If a wrong turn is made, the computer recalculates the route and prompts the driver how to get back on track. These systems are very sophisticated and work wonderfully. Although they are fairly expensive, they are definitely worth considering as a purchase for a driver with VCFS. They eliminate the need to rely on maps, minimize the stress of driving in unfamiliar areas, and provide reassurance to a lost (and anxious) driver. They are available at the major computer stores or on line.

It is also imperative that teenagers understand how to respond in case of an accident. They will need to be coached on their legal rights, exchanging information with the other driver, insurance issues, and how to get help in an emergency. All drivers with VCFS should carry a cell phone with them in the car. They should, however, be taught not to use the phone and drive at the same time.

Finally, the maintenance of the vehicle may need adult supervision. Don't assume that the teenager with VCFS will remember the car needs an oil change or its tires rotated. Another person will need to oversee the repairs and safety checks of the vehicle.

## Social Life

Many parents report difficulties with their teenager's self-esteem and social skills. It is not uncommon for teenagers with VCFS to complain of bullying, teasing, feeling left out of the social mainstream. Perhaps with better interventions in earlier grades, more social problems will be eliminated. However, even with coaching, young adults with VCFS often misread social cues, respond inappropriately in social situations, and are poor social communicators. In addition, their poor planning ability interferes with making and keeping friends, organizing their social calendars, or participating in after-school clubs or activities.

Most teenagers with VCFS will need help with this aspect of their life. Speech and language therapists can help with practicing pragmatic speech. Role playing social situations and helping the teenager better interpret others' intentions is important. It may be necessary to insist that the young adult join one social activity at the high school or to assist him or her in making social plans. Churches and synagogues may have youth group opportunities for high school students to become involved in community projects or social clubs. The summer may also be an opportunity to enhance interaction skills at an overnight or day camp. Encouraging these types of experiences helps these students build skills that enhance interpersonal relationships and improve independent living skills.

## Sex Education

As medicine has improved to treat the heart defects and immune difficulties associated with this syndrome, more and more affected children are surviving into adulthood and childbearing age. It is imperative that young adults understand issues involving both their sexuality and their unique situation regarding their genetic makeup. Students with VCFS have a 50% chance of passing the genetic deletion to a child. As mentioned earlier in the book, there are limited studies on adults with this syndrome. Also of concern is young adults' ability to care properly for a child if they are struggling to acquire academics and life skills themselves. All young adults with this syndrome would benefit from seeing a genetic counselor to help them understand the syndrome and the risks associated with having a child with VCFS. A counselor could also explain medical options available to couples that would allow them to have a healthy baby at some time in the future.

Teachers of sex education classes need to be made aware of the learning differences of students with VCFS, and parents will also need to reinforce the concepts covered in this class as they do for other academic subjects. It is also important for these students to understand the Internet, sexual predators, and the laws that govern behavior in regard to sexual encounters. There is a limited amount of anecdotal evidence that some young adults develop an unhealthy obsession with sexual issues. Sadly, this type of behavior led to an Internet violation and a possible prison term for a young man with VCFS (Baker-Gomaz, 2004). Education staff and parents should take special care to observe the student's computer use and friendship groups. They can then step forward to offer needed guidance and set limits.

## Life Skills

Finally, as stated earlier, studies have shown that young adults with VCFS have poor acquisition of life skills. Many do not learn these common sense tasks without direct instruction. This is the time to emphasize those aspects of daily living such as budgeting, cooking, laundry, filling out forms, job skills, banking, safety around the house, etc. The goal is teaching those tasks that will allow the teenager with VCFS to manage in an apartment (or dorm) away from home and without supervision. Texas School for the Blind has a useful checklist that parents and schools can use to identify all of these independent skills. It can be purchased on line at http://www.tsbvi.edu, under Independent Living Skills Activity Routines. There is a more extensive curriculum also available if the school needs one. A reassessment of these daily living skills would be something to consider for the special education team. Many high schools offer regular education classes in cooking, personal finance, or home/consumer issues. This is also a skill area that can be addressed in a student's individual education plan.

## Legal Considerations and Approaching Adulthood

It is also important that all teenagers with VCFS are given direct instruction in the laws that pertain to them as they approach adulthood. Do not assume that common sense will keep them out of trouble. They often have poor problem-solving skills, lack social awareness, and do not fully understand cause and effect. All teenagers are vulnerable to making poor choices. Young adults with cognitive disabilities are particularly at risk.

Drinking and drug abuse are rampant in high school. In order to fit in, many students take risks and engage in self-destructive behavior. If the teenager with VCFS is on prescription drugs to treat the psychological difficulties associated with this syndrome, drinking and illegal drug use are extremely dangerous. A frank discussion between a treating physician and the teenager with VCFS can be helpful in spelling out the risks involved with substance abuse. Parents and staff need to be very vigilant in monitoring behavior to try to avoid dangerous situations. Supervision and strict rules may be necessary to insure the well-being of a teenager who makes poor choices.

Clearly, there are many considerations to take into account in planning an appropriate educational program for a teenager with VCFS. Parents and educators are urged to meet frequently and to work closely to provide a safe, secure, and nurturing environment at a very vulnerable time the student's life. When life becomes stressful, it is wise to step back and revisit the long-range goal of a mentally healthy, happy, independent adult. With this in mind, a program that emphasizes success, growth, and realistic expectations should be agreeably implemented.

## REFERENCES

Baker-Gomez, S. (2004). *Missing genetic pieces: Strategies for living with VCFS, the chromosome 22q11 deletion*. Phoenix, AZ: Desert Pearl Publisher.

Kok, L. L., & Soloman, R.T. (1995). Velocardiofacial syndrome: Learning difficulties and intervention. *Journal of Medical Genetics, 32*(8), 612–618.

# BIBLIOGRAPHY/SUGGESTED READINGS

Bowen, J. M., Jenson, W. R., & Clark, E. (2004). *School-based interventions for students with behavior problems.* New York: Kluwer Academic/Plenum Publishers.

Cobb, J. (2001). *Learning how to learn: Getting into and surviving college when you have a learning disability.* Washington, DC: CWLA Press.

Flexer, R., Simmons, T., Luft, P., & Baer, R. (2004). *Transition planning for secondary students with disabilities.* Prentice Hall.

Garland, E. J. (1997). *Depression is the pits, but I'm getting better: A guide for adolescents.* Washington, DC: Magination Press.

Hamilton, S. F. (1990). *Apprenticeship for adulthood: Preparing youth for the future.* New York: Free Press.

Larcombe, A. (1985). *Mathematical learning difficulties in the secondary school: Pupil needs and teacher roles.* Milton Keynes UK, Philadelphia, PA: Open University.

Papolos, D., & Papolos, J. (2002). *The bipolar child, The definitive and reassuring guide to childhood's most misunderstood disorder.* Broadway.

Pautler, A. J., & Barlow, M. L. (1990). *Vocational education in the 1990s: Major issues.* Ann Arbor, MI: Prakken Publications.

Pierangelo, R., & Kolstoe, O. (1999). *Transition education services for adolescents with disabilities.* Allen & Bacon.

Prince-Hughes, D. (2002). *Aquamarine blue 5: Personal stories of college students with autism.* Athens, OH: Swallow Press/Ohio University Press.

Sarkees-Wircenski, M., & Scott, J. L. (1995). *Vocational special needs.* Homewood, IL: American Technical Publishers.

Shapiro, J., & Rich, R. (1999). *Facing learning disabilities in the adult years.* New York: Oxford University Press.

Sicile-Kira, C., & Grandin, T. () *Adolescents on the autism spectrum: A parent's guide to the cognitive, social, physical and transition needs of teenagers with autism spectrum disorders.* Perigee Trade.

Solden, S. (2002). *Journeys through ADDulthood: Discover a new sense of identity and meaning while living with attention deficit disorder.* New York: Walker & Co.

Stefan, S. (2001). *Unequal rights: Discrimination against people with mental disabilities and the Americans with Disabilities Act.* Washington, DC: American Psychological Association.

Tomlinson, C. A., & Strickland, C. A. (2005). *Differentiation in practice: A resource guide for differentiating curriculum, grades 9–12.* Alexandria, VA: Association for Supervision and Curriculum Development.

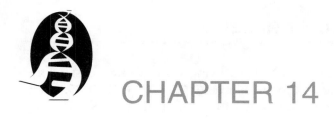

# CHAPTER 14

# Transition to Adulthood (A Model Program)

## *Ages 18–21*

*I*n many ways, this aspect of a disabled student's education can be the most challenging for school districts to address. According to the IDEA law, the public school system is responsible for providing the education and supports to any student with disabilities through the age of 21. At that time, the responsibility for job training shifts to other government agencies such as the Department of Vocational Rehabilitation. *Once a child graduates from high school, the school district is no longer responsible for providing any educational assistance.* Therefore, if students with VCFS graduate with their classmates at age 18, they forfeit their right to any further assistance from the school district, even though they are eligible for an additional three years of service.

Historically, school districts have only provided services through age 21 for their most disabled populations. Some students with VCFS who are labeled as cognitively disabled (IQ less than 70) would easily fall into this group and typically will be offered programming in life skills and job training. Other students with VCFS with higher IQs, however, will likely be graduated with their high school class even though they do *not* possess the skills they need to succeed in a post-secondary training program or in the job market. They do not have skills to allow them to be gainfully employed or the ability to apply independently for government assistance. They will need help with budgeting, banking, locating living accommodations, and applying for jobs.

## CASE VIGNETTE

Mark was a 17-year-old student with VCFS living on the east coast of the United States. He had a typical VCFS profile: FSIQ 77, VIQ 83, PIQ 75, much lower than expected reading comprehension and math scores, difficulty when confronted with complex tasks, difficulty sustaining attention, working memory deficits, significant trouble with problem-solving tasks, language deficits, and slow processing speed. He also demonstrated significant difficulties in managing complex visual/perceptual information. His academic high school plan had included numerous accommodations, but he struggled in all areas. His classes incorporated vocational training in the areas of culinary arts and facilities management, but he experienced difficulty in both settings. Teachers reported that he became overwhelmed and confused with language as well as multidimensional tasks. He had difficulty remembering what was presented in class well enough to complete homework at home.

Despite these learning challenges, the school district intended to graduate Mark at the end of the school year with a certificate of attendance diploma. This action would end the district's responsibility to continue to provide services for Mark until age 21, even though he clearly had not demonstrated that he was capable of gainful employment or of successfully attending a post-secondary education establishment. Mark's parents sought to block his graduation and with the help of an educational consultant knowledgeable about VCFS, they worked with the district to provide a more suitable transition program for him.

When most seniors graduate from high school they plan to attend college or technical school or perhaps join the military. All of these options can be quite daunting to an 18-year-old student with VCFS. Even though colleges and tech schools offer disability services to their students, the level of maturity needed to access these programs may be unrealistic for a young adult with VCFS. Most students with VCFS will likely not have the life skills necessary to live independently in an unsupervised college environment. In addition, those students with VCFS who develop some of the mental health challenges associated with this syndrome will likely find the stress of living away from home and the demands of additional schooling overwhelming.

Young adulthood is also the time when it is really necessary to assess the kinds of supports an adult with VCFS will need throughout his or her lifetime. This can be difficult for parents to face, but it is necessary to put these pieces in place in the event that something would happen to the student's primary caregivers. At age 18 the law assumes that a person is an adult and able to make informed decisions. That person will be held accountable for contracts signed, expenses incurred, and agreements made. Parents must ask themselves, "Will our child be able to manage on his or her own if something happens to us?" If the answer is, "No," they must make plans to secure the needed supports in their community. In the United States, this support can come in the form of financial support (social security, Medicaid, state supplements), vocational (public school system, Department of Vocational Rehabilitation), and life skills support (public schools, Department of Health and Human Services programs for adults with disabilities, guardianships, case management). Parents of children elsewhere can contact their government to determine what kinds of supports are available for disabled adults in their country.

The transition plan for a student age 16 and older should look at all of these areas and make the community contacts necessary to ensure a smooth transition from high school to adult life. The educational team is responsible for contacting these agencies and arranging for meetings to plan how a student's needs will be addressed as the burden of care shifts from the public school system to a system of community-based supports.

Some of the outcomes desired at the time of graduating from high school might include:

- Independent living in an apartment for at least one year with supports to maintain apartment, cook, clean, get own food, etc.

- Reading and math skills at a competitive employment level and at a level needed for chosen career path

- Job/career field solidly chosen after a careful assessment as to whether the job/career is a realistic goal

- Preliminary coursework completed at a technical college or other post-secondary environment and supports clearly in place that will be needed for a successful full-time transition

- Speech, vision, and OT remediation to effectively deal with memory, communication, and perceptual deficits. The desired outcome would be independent functioning.

- Assistive technology identified and in place including a laptop, Palm, visual supports, etc.; also needed is an up-to-date assistive technology assessment to include memory aids

- Basic budgeting and banking/financial skills

- Daily living skills including self-monitoring medication, making and keeping own appointments, etc.

- Binder developed with all necessary numbers and supports in an easily accessible form

- Coordination with all community agencies that would be responsible for job supports, living assistance, etc., and a plan for what is available and who will pay for it

- On-the-job coaching in a competitive employment setting in chosen career

■ Advocacy skills that include understanding VCFS and accommodations needed

■ Skills needed to begin tech school or job training as a full-time student

At age 18, most students with VCFS will not have met these outcomes. These areas can be addressed in a carefully crafted transition program set up through the student's public school.

## A MODEL TRANSITION PROGRAM

The Middleton-Cross Plains Area School District Model Transition Program is one example of how a school district can creatively use resources to address the unique needs of the VCFS population. This program was designed to meet the needs of a 19-year-old student with VCFS who had met the district requirements for high school graduation (completed the required high school classes), but did not have the skills needed to live independently, the ability to advocate well for himself, or the capability to manage his finances. The typical program for students with a cognitive impairment was not appropriate for this student. He had always been in a regular education environment (with supports), independently drove a car, worked with support at a toy store, held a second degree black belt in karate, and had a few typically developing friends. His academic skills ranged from middle school level to high school (for decoding words) and he had good computer and music skills. He was well aware of his VCFS difficulties and he was keenly aware of how others perceived him. He wanted most to fit in to the typical teenage development pattern and resisted anything that would single him out as being "stupid." A transition program consisting of taking life skills classes with a cognitively impaired group of students would not be in this student's best interest and was challenged vigorously by his parents when this program was first offered by the school district. After several meetings, a program uniquely tailored to this student's needs was agreed upon. The student "walked" through the graduation ceremony with his class. He attended the parties, had senior pictures taken, but did *not* receive a diploma. Instead, the next fall he continued to receive remediation services provided by the school district.

The first year of the transition program:

■ Student met daily for one-on-one tutoring help in math and reading skills with his case manager at a site off of the high school campus. This occurred at the district administrative center, which helped avoid any embarrassment the student would feel attending class at the high school.

Foreign language instruction, middle school, 188–189
Fragile X syndrome, viii, ix–xi
Freedom from Distractibility (WISC III), 22
Functional Assessment and Intervention System (FAIS), 29

**G**

Gates-MacGinitie Reading Tests, 167
Genetics
    and diagnosis, 12
    distinct diseases, 4
    evaluation referral, 11–12, 64
    mental disorder/genetic link, 8
    nomenclature, 7
    and phenotypes, 9
    and schizophrenia risk, 63
    of syndromes, 4
    understanding of, vii
    variable expression, 9–10
    VCFS and ADHD, 43
    VCFS history, 5–6, 8
Genome, vii, 8, 12
Goldman-Fristoe Test of Articulation-2, 87
Graves' disease, 101
Gray, Carol, 153
Gray Oral Reading Test 4, 167
Gray Silent Reading Test, 167
Greenes, Carole, 171
Gross motor activities, 174–175
Guilford, J. P., 163

**H**

Handwriting accommodations, 220–221
Head Start Performance Standards, 123
Health and Human Services Department, 207
High school (ages 14–18). *See also main heading* Accommodations
    academics, 197–199
    case study, 195–196
    cell phones, 200
    college prep consideration, 194
    computers, 186
    direct instruction, 198–199
    drinking, 202
    driving instruction, 199–200
    drug abuse, 202
    independence development, 198
    job experience courses, 197
    legal considerations, 200, 202
    life skills, 201–202
    one-on-one settings, 198
    organizational assistance, 197–198
    overview, 193–194, 193–202
    preferential classroom seating, 198
    public *versus* private, 195
    rote memory strategies, 198
    scaffolding, 198
    sex education, 201
    small group settings, 198
    social life, 200–201
    study guide provision, 198
    technical school options, 195
    vocational training, 196–197
History, VCFS, vii–viii, 4–8
Hole-in-the-Wall Gang Camps, 189
Holoprosencephaly sequence, 7
Home–school communication accommodations, 220
How Does Your Engine Run? The Alert Program for Self-Regulation, 138, 154
Hubert, Bill, 154
Human Genome Project, vii, 8
Hyperthyroidism, 101
Hypotonia, 20–21

**I**

I CAN Learn Mathematics Curriculum, 186
IDEA (Individuals with Disabilities Education Act), 120, 211
Identification, 10
IEP (individualized education plans), 80–82, 183, 195
Illness, childhood
    autoimmune disease, 101
    bronchitis, 99
    croup, 99
    ear infection, 98
    fevers, 99–100
    gastrointestinal complaints, 101

Illness, childhood *(continued)*
and hypotonia, 101–102
low body temperature, 99–100
LRI (lower respiratory tract
infections), 99
malaise, 101
pneumonia, 99
seizures, 101
sinus infection, 98
and surgical repair, 100
tonsillitis, 98
URI (upper respiratory infections),
97–99
VCFS immune system compromises,
95–97
Individualized education plans (IEP),
80–82, 183, 195
Individuals with Disabilities Education
Act (IDEA), 120, 211
Institute of Education Sciences, U.S.
Department of Education,
185–186
Interact history simulations, 173
Interactive Computer-Aided Natural
Learning, 186
Intervention, educational. *See also main
heading* Accommodations
birth to 3 programs, 117–118
case management, 137–138
CBA (curriculum based assessment),
114, 115
CBM (curriculum-based
measurement), 114, 115
classroom environmental needs,
136–138
elementary grades 3–5 (ages 8–11),
159–176 *(See also main heading*
Elementary grades 3–5 [ages
8–11])
format considerations, 135–136
high school (ages 14–18), 193–202
*(See also main heading*
Accommodations; High school
[ages 14–18] *for details*)
Kindergarten–second grade (ages
5–7), 143–156 *(See also main
heading* Accommodations;
Kindergarten–second grade [ages
5–7] *for details*)

middle school (ages 11–14), 179–189
*(See also main entry*
Accommodations; *entry* Middle
school [ages 11–14])
performance assessment, 115
portfolio assessment, 114
preschool (ages 3–5), 119–132 *(See also
main entry* Accommodations;
*entry* Preschool intervention
[ages 3–5] *for details*)
reading, 144–148
selecting between educational
formats, 135–139
sensory integration, 138–139
and Smart Board systems, 136–137
IQ measurement, 30–31, 121–122
IQ subnormalcy
decline with age, 120
reasons for, 40–41
testing caveats, 30–31
and VSD and cleft palate, 11 *(See also*
Cognition)

**K**

Kaufman Assessment Battery for
Children, 2nd ed. (KABC-11),
28
Kindergarten–second grade (ages 5–7).
*See also main heading*
Accommodations
automaticity attainment, 150
Bal-A-Vix-X: Rhythmic, Balance/
Auditory/Vision Exercises for
Brain and Brain-Body Integration,
154
basal reading approach, 147
behavior issues, 154
*The Berenstain Bears and the Messy
Room* (Stan & Jan Berenstain),
148
and classification, 149
On Cloud Nine program, 150
comprehension monitoring, 146
and computers, 146–147, 149
computer screen reading, 147
cooperative learning, 146
and feedback/guidance, 145
health concerns, 154

How Does Your Engine Run? The Alert Program for Self-Regulation, 154
and kinesiology, 154
Kumon math and reading program, 150–151
life/social skills, 153
mathematics, 149–152
memory assistance, 148
number conservation, 149
number sense understanding, 149–150
Number Worlds, 150
occupational therapy, 155
one-to-one correspondence of things, 149
one-to-one settings, 147
oral communication, 148–149
ordering sequentially, 149
organizers, graphic/semantic, 146
*The Original Social Stories Book* (gray), 153
overview, 143–144
phonemic awareness, 144–145
phonics, 145
question answering/generation, 146
reading, 144–148
Reading Street program, 147
real-world applications, 152
remedial strategies, 150
science, 152
self-regulation, 154
Singapore Math, 150
small group settings, 147
social stories, 153
social studies, 152
spelling, 148–149
story structure instruction, 146
summarization skill teaching, 146
time allotment, 147
vocabulary instruction, 145–146
writing, 148–149
Kinesiology, 154
Kumon program, 151, 166, 187

**L**

Language education, 19–20
Language skills, 77

Learning issues overview, 25–28
Life skills
elementary grades 3–5 (ages 8–11), 175–176
high school (ages 14–18), 201–202
testing, 29–30

**M**

Marcy, Steve and Janis, 186
Marion, Robert W., 6
Mastropieri, M. A., 184
Mathematics education, 18–19, 45–47
elementary grades 3–5 (ages 8–11), 170–172
Kindergarten–second grade (ages 5–7), 149–152
middle school (ages 11–14), 185–187
preschool intervention (ages 3–5), 127–130
preschool readiness, 127–130
Medicaid, 207
Medications, 215
Depakote, 67
mood stabilizers, 67
Prozac, 67
psychiatric, 67–68
Ritalin, 67
serotonin-specific reuptake inhibitors (SSRI), 67
side effects, negative, 67
stimulant, 67
Memory
executive function, 21–22
overview, 21
visual-spatial, 21, 40
working memory, 21–22, 160–163, 168–169, 182–185, 222–223
Memory Matrix computer program, 163
Mentoring programs, 66, 165–166
Middle school (ages 11–14). *See also main heading* Accommodations
academics, 182–189
acrostic techniques, 184
algebra, 186–187
arts classes, 188–189
away-from-home experience, 189
Camp Kodiak, 189

Middle school (ages 11–14) *(continued)*
  cognitive remediation therapy,
    183–185
  Cognitive Tutor, 186
  communication skills, 181–182
  Comprehensive Reading Intervention
    Solution, 187
  dress, 180–181
  Fast ForWord, 187
  foreign language instruction, 188–189
  grooming, 180–181
  health education, 180–181
  Hole-in-the-Wall Gang Camps, 189
  I CAN Learn Mathematics Curriculum,
    186
  Interactive Computer-Aided Natural
    Learning, 186
  keyword memory technique, 184
  Kumon reading program, 187
  language skills, 181–182
  mathematics, 185–187
  *Middle School Math with Pizzazz*
    (Marcy & Marcy), 186
  mnemonic techniques, 183–184
  occupational therapy, 185
  one-on-one settings, 187–188
  overview, 179–180
  peg words memory technique, 184
  pre-algebra, 186
  preteaching, 187–188
  process recording, 187
  reading, 187–188
  Read 180 program, 187
  reteaching, 188
  science, 188
  small group setting, 187–188
  social studies, 188
  summer camp, 189
  templates use, 183
  Victory Junction Camp, 189
  visual perceptual impairment
    accommodations, 185
  What Works Clearinghouse, 185–186
  working memory, 182–185
*Middle School Math with Pizzazz*
    (Marcy & Marcy), 186
Motor abilities
  delays, 51–52

NEPSY battery, 20
  overview, 20–21
Motor/visual accomodations, 220–221
Music lessons, 175

**N**

NAEYC (National Association for the
    Education of Young Children),
    123
National Reading Panel, 144, 146
NEPSY battery, 20, 29, 30
1992 reports, 8
No Child Left Behind (NCLB), 172
Nonverbal learning disability (NVLD),
    31–32, 224–226
Notetaking accommodations, 222
Number Worlds program, 129, 150, 171
NVLD (nonverbal learning disability),
    31–32, 224–226

**O**

Obsessive-compulsive disorder. *See* OCD
    (obsessive-compulsive disorder)
Occupational therapy (OT)
  adult transition, 207
  Kindergarten–second grade (ages
    5–7), 32, 155
  middle school (ages 11–14), 185
  preschool intervention (ages 3–5), 32,
    126–127
OCD (obsessive-compulsive disorder)
  case study, 61–62, 64–65
  incidence with VCFS, 60
  medication, 67
On Cloud Nine math program, 129–130,
    150, 171
Optimism, 215
Organization accommodations, 218–219
*The Original Social Stories Book*
    (Gray), 153
OT. *See* occupational therapy (OT)

**P**

Parents
  guidance treatment, 66–67

home practice, 83–84, 85
math readiness instruction, 130
and psychiatric issues, 66–67
selecting between educational
    formats, 135–139
tutor hiring, 165, 166
Patent ductus arteriosus (PDA), 10
PDA (patent ductus arteriosus), 10
Peabody Development of Motor Skills,
    21
Performance assessment, 115
Phenotypes of VCFS, 9
Phobias, 61–62
Phonemic awareness
    Kindergarten–second grade (ages
      5–7), 144–145
    preschool intervention (ages 3–5),
      131
Phonics, 145
Phonological Awareness Test (PAT),
    90–91
PLAI (Preschool Language Assessment
    Instrument-2), 78
Portfolio assessment, 114
Potter sequence, 7
Prader-Willi syndrome, 60
Preschool intervention (ages 3–5). *See
    also main heading*
    Accommodations
    behavior issues, 131–132
    child-focused, 124–126
    and dyscalculia, 128–130
    guidelines, 123–126
    intelligibility reinforcement, 126
    learning environments, 123–124
    maintaining a routine, 127
    math readiness instruction, 127–130
      Building Blocks software, 129
      On Cloud Nine math program,
        129–130
      deficit addressing, 128
      dual coding, 130
      linguistic element teaching, 129
      manipulative use, 129
      model building, 129
      Number Worlds program, 129
      parent intervention, 130
      problem areas, 128

      Singapore Math, 130
      verbalizing solution routes, 130
    occupational therapy, 126–127
    phonemic awareness instruction, 131
    readiness to learn activities, 123–127
    skill modeling/practice, 127
    social relationship building, 126
    special educational referral, 119–121
    transition planning, 127
    using calm voice, 127
    VCFS specifics, 126–127
Preschool Language Assessment
    Instrument-2 (PLAI), 78
Prozac, 67
Psychiatric issues
    ADHD (attention deficit hyperactivity
      disorder), 60, 64–65, 67
    in adolescence, 63–64
    affective disorders, 62–63
    anxiety disorders, 62–63
    assertiveness lack, 58–59
    autism spectrum disorder, 23–24, 58
    bipolar disorder, 23
    case studies, 61–63, 64–65
    depression, 25, 62–63
    low self-esteem, 59
    OCD (obsessive-compulsive disorder),
      60
    overview, 23–24, 57–58
    phobias, 61–62
    predisposition to, 59
    psychosis,
      subthreshold, 63–64
    schizophrenia, 23, 57
    separation anxiety disorder, 64–65
    social skill deficits, 58–59
    stereotypic behaviors, 60
    treatment,
      CBT (cognitive behavioral therapy),
        65
      group social skills training, 65–66
      mentoring program, 66
      parent guidance, 66–67
      social skills training, group, 65–66

**Q**

Questionnaire, Teacher Awareness, ix–xi

# R

Reading education, 19
  elementary grades 3–5 (ages 8–11),
    166–169
  Kindergarten–second grade (ages
    5–7), 144–148
  middle school (ages 11–14), 187–188
Reading Street program, 147
Read 180 program, 187
Receptive One-Word Picture Vocabulary
  Test (ROWPVT), 78, 87
*Research-Based Methods of Reading
  Instruction, Grades K-3* (Vaughn
  & Linan-Thompson), 146
Rey-Osterrieth Complex Figure Test, 29
Rheumatoid arthritis, juvenile, 101
Ritalin, 67
Robin sequence, 7
ROWPVT (Receptive One-Word Picture
  Vocabulary Test), 78, 87

# S

Scales of Independent Behavior-Revised
  (SIB-R), 30
Schizo-affective disorder, 64–65
Schizophrenia, 25, 57, 63
School Behavior Scales (SSBS), 29
School–home communication
  accommodations, 220
Schulman, Linda, 171
Science
  elementary grades 3–5 (ages 8–11),
    172–174
  Kindergarten–second grade (ages
    5–7), 152
  middle school (ages 11–14), 188
Screening, 10–12
Scruggs, T. E., 184
Self-esteem, 59
Separation anxiety disorder case study,
  64–65
Serotonin-specific reuptake inhibitors
  (SSRI), 67
Shellenberger, Sherry, 138
Shprintzen, Robert, vii
SIB-R (Scales of Independent Behavior-
  Revised), 30

Singapore Math, 130, 150, 171
SLP (speech-language pathologists)
  expressive/receptive language skills,
    148–149
  school,
    middle school (ages 11–14), 181
  school-based (*See also* Speech-
    language therapy)
  and screening, 10
Social Security, 207, 209, 211
Social skills
  case study, 61–62
  detailed, 58–59
  group training, 65–66
Social Skills Rating Scales (SSRS), 30
Social studies
  elementary grades 3–5 (ages 8–11),
    172–174
  Kindergarten–second grade (ages
    5–7), 152
  middle school (ages 11–14), 188
SOI (Structure of Intellect System),
  162–163
Spatiotemporal representation, 21
Speech
  intelligibility, 76–77
  voice,
    articulation, 74–77, 230–231
    "cleft palate" speech, 75–77
    fluency, 77
    phonological disorder, 75
    pitch, 73
    quality, 72
    resonance, 73–74
    and tonsil hypertorphy, 74
    treatment, 73
    volume, 73
    VPI (velopharyngeal insufficiency),
      74, 76–77
Speech-language pathologists. *See* SLP
  (speech-language pathologists)
Speech-language therapy. *See also*
  Intervention, educational
  preschool, 77–78
  school,
    articulation therapy, 83
    direct instruction, 83–84
    and home practice, 83–84, 85

IEP (individualized education plans), 80–82, 183
overview, 78–79
procedures, 82–83
service model, 81–82
services qualification, 79–80, 84, 85–93, 119–121
Speech therapy. *See also* Intervention, educational
articulation, 19, 83
conversational style, 20
expressive language, 20
phonological disorders, 75
pragmatic language, 20
receptive language, 19
voice treatment, 73
Spungin, Rika, 171
SSBS (School Behavior Scales), 29
SSRI (serotonin-specific reuptake inhibitors), 67
SSRS (Social Skills Rating Scales), 30
Standardized Reading Inventory 2, 167
Stanford-Binet Intelligence Scale, 4th ed., 28
Strong, W. B., 5–6
Structure of Intellect System (SOI), 162–163
Summer camp, 189
Supplemental Security Income (SSI), 211
Surgery
for anatomical abnormalities, 100–101

**T**

TAPS-3 (Test of Auditory Processing Skills), 88–90
TCC (Token Test for Children), 78
Teacher Awareness Questionnaire, ix–xi
Teacher exercises, 229–234
Teacher knowledge, viii, ix–xi
Teasing, 175
Testing
ABAS (Adaptive Behavior Assessment System), 30
Achenbach System of Empirically Based Assessment, 29
of achievement, 28–29

ADI-R (Autism Diagnostic Interview-Revised), 30
ADOS (Autism Diagnostic Observation Schedule), 30
of attention, 29
BASC (Behavior Assessment System for Children), 29
Bayley Scale, 17
of behavior, 29
BISD-II (Bayley Scales of Infant Development, 2nd edition), 17, 28
BISD-III (Bayley Scales of Infant Development, 3rd edition), 17, 28
Bruininks-Orseretsky Test of Motor Proficiency, 21
caveats, 30–31
CBCL (Child Behavior Checklist), 29
CELF (Clinical Evaluation of Language Fundamentals), 30
CELF-P (ages Clinical Evaluation of Language Functions-Preschool), 78
cognitive, 16–18, 28, 30–31
Comprehensive Reading Assessment Battery, 167
CPT (Continuous Performance Test-II), 29
CRS-R (Connors Rating Scales-Revised), 29
CTOPP (Comprehensive Test of Phonological Processing), 145
CVLT (California Verbal Learning, Test), 30
DIBELS (Dynamic Indicators of Basic Early Literacy Skills), 145
EOWPVT (Expressive One-Word Picture Vocabulary Test), 78, 88, 91
FAIS (Functional Assessment and Intervention System), 29
Freedom from Distractibility (WISC III), 22
Gates-MacGinitie Reading Tests, 167
Goldman-Fristoe Test of Articulation-2, 87
Gray Oral Reading Test 4, 167

Testing *(continued)*
Gray Silent Reading Test, 167
KABC-11 (Kaufman Assessment
Battery for Children, 2nd ed.), 28
of language, 30
of life/social skills, 29–30
NEPSY battery, 20, 29, 30
neurocognitive, 27–28
neuropsychological, 16
PAT (Phonological Awareness Test),
90–91
Peabody Development of Motor Skills,
21
PLAI (ages Preschool Language
Assessment Instrument-2), 78
of problem solving, 29
Rey-Osterrieth Complex Figure Test,
29
ROWPVT (Receptive One-Word
Picture Vocabulary Test), 78, 87
SIB-R (Scales of Independent
Behavior-Revised), 30
of social/life skills, 29–30
of speech, 30
SSBS (School Behavior Scales), 29
SSRS (Social Skills Rating Scales), 30
Standardized Reading Inventory 2,
167
Stanford-Binet Intelligence Scale, 4th
ed., 28
TAPS-3 (Test of Auditory Processing
Skills), 88–90, 90
Test of Reading Comprehension, 167
TOLD (Test of Language
Development), 30
TOPA (Test of Phonological
Awareness), 145
TOPL (Test of Pragmatic Language),
30
TOPS (Test of Problem Solving), 29
TOWL (Test of Written Language-III),
30
TTC (Token Test for Children), 78, 90
VABS (Vineland Adaptive Behavior
Scales), 29
Verbal Comprehension Index (WISC
III), 22
of visual perception, 29

VMI (Beery-Tuktenica Developmental
Test of Visual-Motor Integration),
29
WAIS (Wechsler Adult Intelligence
Scale), 122
WIAT-II (Wechsler Individual
Achievement Test, 2nd ed.), 28
WISC III (Wechsler Intelligence Scale
for Children), 22
WISC IV (Wechsler Intelligence Scale
for Children, 4th ed.), 28
Wisconsin Card Sorting Task, 29
Woodcock Johnson Test of
Achievement III, 29
Woodcock Reading Mastery, 167
Word-R Test, 91–92
WPPSI-R (ages Wechsler Preschool
and Primary Scale of
Intelligence), 17, 28
WRAT (Wide Range Achievement
Test), 18
Yopp-Singer Test of Phoneme
Segmentation, 145
Testing accommodations, 219–220
Test of Auditory Processing Skills (TAPS-
3), 88–90
Test of Language Development (TOLD),
30
Test of Phonological Awareness (TOPA),
145
Test of Pragmatic Language (TOPL), 30
Test of Problem Solving (TOPS), 29
Test of Written Language-III (TOWL), 30
Test writing
accommodations, 219–220
Tetralogy of Fallot (TOF)
case study, 62–63
as screening basis, 10
surgical repair, 4
The Thinker Math program, 171–172
TOF. *See* Tetralogy of Fallot
Token Test for Children (TCC), 78
Token Test for Children (TTC), 90
TOLD (Test of Language Development),
30
TOPA (Test of Phonological Awareness),
145
TOPL (Test of Pragmatic Language), 30

TOWL (Test of Written Language-III), 30
Treatment
    CBT (cognitive behavioral therapy),
        65
    group social skills training, 65–66
    medications, 67–68
    mentoring program, 66
    parent guidance, 66–67
    social skills training, group, 65–66
TTC (Token Test for Children), 90
22q11.2 deletion. *See also* VCFS (velo-
    cardio-facial syndrome)
    delays with, 15
    and FISH screening, vii, 10
    prevalence, viii

**V**

VABS (Vineland Adaptive Behavior
    Scales), 29
VCFS (velo-cardio-facial syndrome). *See
    also* 22q11.2 deletion
    attention problems, 41–44
    brain imaging studies, 40–41
    characteristics, 9
    de novo, 17
    diagnosis, viii, 12, 39–40
    fact sheet, 102–110
    familial, 17
    future, 12
    history, vii–viii, 4–8
    immune system compromises, 95–97
    name coinage, 4–5
    phenotypes, 9
    present state, 8–12
    prevalence, viii
    Teacher Awareness Questionnaire,
        ix–xi
Velo-Cardio-Facial Syndrome Educational
    Foundation, Inc., viii, 7, 180–181
Velopharyngeal insufficiency (VPI), 74,
    76–77
Verbal Comprehension Index (WISC III),
    22
Victory Junction Camp, 189
Vineland Adaptive Behavior Scales
    (VABS), 29
Visual-Motor Integration test (VMI), 29

Visual-spatial impairment
    and education, 18
    face recognition, 48–50
    and mathematics, 18, 45–47
    memory, 21, 40
    object recognition, 48–50
VMI (Visual-Motor Integration test), 29
Vocational Rehabilitation Department,
    207
VPI (velopharyngeal insufficiency), 74,
    76–77
VSD (ventriculoseptal defect), 4, 10, 11

**W**

WAIS (Wechsler Adult Intelligence
    Scale), 122
Web sites
    Comprehensive Reading Intervention
        Solution, 187
    Fast ForWord program, 166
    Highsmith supplies, 173
    Kumon program, 151
    *Middle School Math with Pizzazz*
        (Marcy & Marcy), 186
    Social Security Administration, 211
    Structure of Intellect System (SOI),
        162–163
    test publishers, 28–30
    The Thinker Math program, 171
    What Works Clearinghouse, 185–186
Wechsler Adult Intelligence Scale
    (WAIS), 122
Wechsler Individual Achievement Test,
    2nd ed. (WIAT-II), 28
Wechsler Intelligence Scale for Children
    (WISC III), 22
Wechsler Preschool and Primary Scale
    of Intelligence (WPPSI-R), 17, 28
*What Does Everybody Else Know That
    I Don't? Social Skills Help for
    Adults With Attention
    Deficit/Hyperactivity Disorder*
    (Novotni & Peterson), 180
What Works Clearinghouse, 185–186
Wide Range Achievement Test (WRAT),
    18
Williams, Mary Sue, 138

Williams syndrome, 60
WISC III (Verbal Comprehension Index), 22
WISC III (Wechsler Intelligence Scale for Children), 22
WISC IV Wechsler Intelligence Scale for Children, 4th ed.), 28
Wisconsin Card Sorting Task, 29
Woodcock Johnson Test of Achievement III, 29
Woodcock Reading Mastery, 167
Word-R Test, 91–92
Working memory accommodations, 222–223

WPPSI-R (Wechsler Preschool and Primary Scale of Intelligence), 17, 28
WRAT (Wide Range Achievement Test), 18

**Y**

Yopp-Singer Test of Phoneme Segmentation, 145

**Z**

Zellweger syndrome, 7